HOMEMADE LIQUID SOAP MAKING

A Complete Guide for Crafting Organic and Natural Liquid Soap: Step-by-Step Recipes, Essential Oils, Marketing Strategies, and Eco-Friendly Techniques All Included.

Eddie R. Melvin

TABLE OF CONTENT

CHAPTER ONE

INTRODUCTION TO LIQUID SOAP MAKING

1.1. History and Benefits of Liquid Soap

Liquid soap has an intriguing history that traces back to the earliest human civilizations. People have always needed to clean themselves and their surroundings, but the methods and ingredients they used have evolved dramatically over the centuries.

In ancient times, people discovered that mixing ashes with fats created a substance that could clean almost anything. These early soaps were rudimentary but effective. As time went on, the art of soap making became more refined. In the Middle Ages, soap makers began using more sophisticated techniques and ingredients, such as animal fats and plant ashes. The process was labor-intensive and often kept as a closely guarded secret within families or guilds.

The real game-changer came in the 19th century when the industrial revolution allowed for the mass production of soap. This made soap more accessible to the general public, improving hygiene standards across the board. However, it wasn't until the 20th century that liquid soap made its debut. The first liquid soap was patented in 1865 by William Sheppard, but it wasn't widely adopted until much later. In the 1980s, liquid soap started to become a household staple, thanks to its convenience and the growing popularity of hand pumps.

Today, liquid soap is everywhere. It's found in kitchens, bathrooms, hospitals, and offices. Its rise to prominence is largely due to its numerous benefits:

1. Hygiene and Convenience Liquid soap is often seen as more hygienic than bar soap. Because it's dispensed in small, controlled amounts, it reduces the risk of spreading germs between users. This makes it an ideal choice for public restrooms and communal spaces.

2. Customizability One of the biggest advantages of liquid soap is its versatility. You can easily customize it with different fragrances, colors, and additional ingredients like moisturizers or antibacterial agents. This means you can tailor your soap to meet specific needs, whether it's a soothing lavender scent for a relaxing hand wash or a citrus-infused formula for a refreshing shower gel.

3. Skin Benefits Many liquid soaps are formulated to be gentle on the skin, incorporating ingredients like aloe vera, glycerin, and essential oils. These additives can provide moisturizing benefits and help maintain the skin's natural barrier. For people with sensitive skin or specific dermatological conditions, liquid soap can be a much better option than traditional bar soap.

4. Environmentally Friendly Options With growing environmental awareness, there are now many eco-friendly liquid soaps available. These are made with biodegradable ingredients and packaged in recyclable materials. Some companies even offer refill stations to reduce plastic waste, making it easier to be kind to the planet while staying clean.

5. Economic and Efficient Liquid soap can be more economical in the long run. With a controlled dispenser, you're less likely to use more than you need, reducing wastage. Additionally, liquid soap often lasts longer than a bar of soap, especially in households with multiple users.

The journey of liquid soap from its humble beginnings to its current ubiquitous presence is a testament to human ingenuity and our ongoing quest for cleanliness and convenience. Whether you're a seasoned soap maker or a curious beginner, understanding the history and benefits of liquid soap provides a solid foundation for diving into the world of soap making. It's not just about getting clean; it's about creating a product that can be tailored to your exact needs and preferences, offering a personalized touch to everyday hygiene.

1.2. Understanding the Basics of Soap Making

Soap making is a fascinating blend of science and art, a process that transforms simple ingredients into a versatile cleaning product. To truly appreciate the craft, it's important to understand the basic principles behind it. Here, we'll delve into the essential components and steps involved in making soap, focusing on the liquid variety.

The Science of Saponification

At the heart of soap making is a chemical reaction known as saponification. This reaction occurs when fats or oils come into contact with an alkali. For liquid soap, the alkali used is potassium hydroxide (KOH), whereas bar soap typically uses sodium hydroxide (NaOH).

Here's a simplified version of the process:

- ✓ **Fats and Oils**: These are the primary ingredients in soap. They can come from various sources, including vegetable oils (like olive, coconut, and castor oils) and animal fats (such as tallow or lard). Each type of fat or oil contributes different properties to the final product. For example, coconut oil creates a bubbly lather, while olive oil adds moisturizing qualities.

✓ **Alkali (Potassium Hydroxide)**: This substance is crucial for the saponification process. When mixed with fats or oils, it breaks down their molecules, forming soap and glycerin. Glycerin is a natural moisturizer, making it a valuable byproduct of the soap-making process.

The Ingredients

To make liquid soap, you'll need a few basic ingredients:

✓ **Oils and Fats**: As mentioned, these can vary widely. Common choices for liquid soap include olive oil, coconut oil, and castor oil. Each brings unique characteristics to the soap.

✓ **Potassium Hydroxide (KOH)**: This is the alkali used to turn the oils into soap. It's essential to use potassium hydroxide for liquid soap, as sodium hydroxide will result in a solid bar soap.

HOMEMADE LIQUID SOAP MAKING

- ✓ **Distilled Water**: Water is used to dissolve the potassium hydroxide and to dilute the soap paste into a liquid form.

- ✓ **Additives**: These can include fragrance oils, essential oils, colorants, and other beneficial ingredients like aloe vera or vitamin E. Additives allow you to customize your soap to suit your preferences and needs.

The Equipment

The tools required for soap making are relatively simple, but some are essential for safety and accuracy:

- ✓ **Safety Gear**: Gloves, goggles, and an apron are crucial for protecting yourself when handling potassium hydroxide, which is caustic and can cause burns.

- ✓ **Heat-Resistant Containers**: You'll need sturdy containers for mixing and heating your ingredients.

- ✓ **A Stick Blender**: This helps to speed up the saponification process by thoroughly mixing the oils and alkali.

HOMEMADE LIQUID SOAP MAKING

- ✓ **A Slow Cooker or Double Boiler**: These are used to gently heat the soap mixture during the cooking phase.

- ✓ **Measuring Tools**: Accurate measurements are crucial in soap making. Use a digital scale to weigh your ingredients, and measuring spoons and cups for smaller quantities.

The Process

1. **Preparing the Lye Solution**:

   - ✓ Carefully measure and dissolve the potassium hydroxide in distilled water. This step generates heat and should be done in a well-ventilated area with appropriate safety gear. Always add the potassium hydroxide to the water, not the other way around, to prevent splashing.

2. **Mixing Oils and Lye Solution**:

   - ✓ Measure your oils and warm them in a heat-resistant container. Once they reach the right temperature, slowly add the lye solution to the oils while stirring continuously.

3. **Reaching Trace**:

    ✓ Use a stick blender to mix the oils and lye solution until you reach "trace." Trace is the point where the mixture thickens to a pudding-like consistency and leaves a trail when dripped from the blender.

4. **Cooking the Soap**:

    ✓ Pour the mixture into a slow cooker or double boiler and cook on low heat. Stir occasionally and cook until the soap reaches the gel phase and becomes translucent. This process can take several hours.

5. **Diluting the Soap**:

    ✓ Once the soap paste is fully cooked, it needs to be diluted with water to achieve the desired consistency. This step can take some time, and you may need to adjust the amount of water to get the right thickness.

6. **Adding Final Touches**:

    ✓ After dilution, you can add fragrance oils, essential oils, or colorants to your soap. Stir well to ensure even distribution of these additives.

7. **Bottling the Soap**:

   ✓ Once the soap has cooled and reached the desired consistency, pour it into bottles for storage. Properly label your soap and keep it out of reach of children and pets.

Safety First

Safety is paramount when making soap, especially when handling lye. Always wear protective gear and work in a well-ventilated area. Keep vinegar on hand to neutralize any lye spills, and never leave the soap-making process unattended.

Understanding these basics provides a solid foundation for exploring the world of liquid soap making. With practice, you can experiment with different oils, additives, and techniques to create your own unique soaps tailored to your preferences and needs.

1.3. Overview of the Liquid Soap-Making Process

Making liquid soap can seem complex at first glance, but breaking it down into manageable steps makes it easier to understand and execute. Here's an overview of the liquid soap-making process from start to finish.

Step 1: Gather Your Ingredients and Equipment

Before you start, make sure you have all your ingredients and equipment ready. Organization is key to a smooth soap-making experience.

Ingredients:

- ✓ Oils and fats (e.g., olive oil, coconut oil, castor oil)

- ✓ Potassium hydroxide (KOH)

- ✓ Distilled water

- ✓ Fragrance oils or essential oils (optional)

- ✓ Colorants (optional)

Equipment:

- ✓ Safety gear (gloves, goggles, apron)

- ✓ Heat-resistant containers

- ✓ Stick blender

HOMEMADE LIQUID SOAP MAKING

✓ Slow cooker or double boiler

✓ Measuring tools (digital scale, measuring cups and spoons)

Step 2: Prepare the Lye Solution

Safety first! Put on your gloves, goggles, and apron. Work in a well-ventilated area.

1. Measure the required amount of distilled water and pour it into a heat-resistant container.

2. Carefully weigh the potassium hydroxide. Slowly add the potassium hydroxide to the water (never the other way around) while stirring gently. The mixture will heat up and release fumes, so be cautious.

Step 3: Measure and Heat the Oils

1. Measure your oils using a digital scale. Common oils for liquid soap include olive oil for moisturizing properties, coconut oil for lather, and castor oil for a rich texture.

2. Combine the oils in a heat-resistant container and warm them gently. You can use a microwave or a

double boiler to reach the desired temperature, typically around 120°F to 130°F (49°C to 54°C).

Step 4: Combine the Lye Solution and Oils

1. Once the oils are at the right temperature, slowly pour the lye solution into the oils while stirring continuously.

2. Use a stick blender to mix the oils and lye solution until you reach "trace." Trace is when the mixture thickens and leaves a trail when dripped from the blender. This usually takes a few minutes of blending.

Step 5: Cook the Soap Paste

1. Transfer the traced mixture into a slow cooker or double boiler set on low heat.

2. Cook the soap mixture, stirring occasionally. The mixture will go through various stages: it will first become thick like pudding, then go through a gel

phase, and finally become translucent. This process can take several hours.

Step 6: Dilute the Soap Paste

1. Once the soap paste is fully cooked and translucent, it's time to dilute it. This step transforms the thick soap paste into liquid soap.

2. Gradually add distilled water to the soap paste. The amount of water needed will vary based on your recipe and desired soap thickness. Stir well to ensure the soap paste dissolves completely. This can take several hours to a few days.

Step 7: Add Fragrance, Color, and Other Additives

1. After the soap is fully diluted and cooled to room temperature, you can add fragrance oils or essential oils. The amount will depend on your preference and the strength of the oils.

2. If you want to add colorants, do so at this stage. Mix well to ensure even distribution.

3. Other additives, like aloe vera gel or vitamin E, can also be added for additional skin benefits.

Step 8: Bottle and Label Your Soap

HOMEMADE LIQUID SOAP MAKING

1. Once the soap has reached the desired consistency and all additives are thoroughly mixed, it's time to bottle it.

2. Pour the liquid soap into clean, dry bottles. Using a funnel can make this process easier and less messy.

3. Label your bottles with the type of soap, ingredients, and any special instructions. Proper labeling is especially important if you plan to sell or gift your soap.

Final Tips

✓ **Testing and Adjustments**: Test the pH of your soap before using it. Ideally, it should be between 8 and 10. If it's too high, you can dilute it further. If it's too low, the soap may not be fully saponified and could be harsh on the skin.

✓ **Storage**: Store your liquid soap in a cool, dry place. Properly stored, it can last up to a year or more.

✓ **Experimentation**: Don't be afraid to experiment with different oils, fragrances, and additives. Soap making is both a science and an art, allowing for endless creativity and personalization.

By following these steps, you can successfully make your own liquid soap at home. With practice, you'll gain confidence and be able to create a variety of liquid soaps tailored to your preferences and needs. Happy soap making!

CHAPTER TWO

INGREDIENTS AND EQUIPMENT

2.1. Essential Ingredients

Embarking on the journey of making liquid soap at home is both exciting and rewarding. However, before diving into the process, it's crucial to understand the essential ingredients that you'll need. Each component plays a specific role in the creation of your liquid soap, contributing to its cleansing power, texture, scent, and overall quality. Let's break down these ingredients in detail.

Oils and Fats

Oils and fats are the backbone of any soap recipe. They determine the soap's lather, moisturizing properties, and texture. Here's a closer look at some commonly used oils and their benefits:

HOMEMADE LIQUID SOAP MAKING

1. **Olive Oil**:

    ✓ **Properties**: Olive oil is rich in antioxidants and has excellent moisturizing properties. It's gentle on the skin, making it ideal for people with sensitive skin or those prone to dryness.

    ✓ **Role in Soap**: Olive oil creates a mild, creamy lather and contributes to the soap's moisturizing qualities.

2. **Coconut Oil**:

    ✓ **Properties**: Coconut oil is well-known for its ability to produce a rich, bubbly lather. It also has natural antibacterial and antifungal properties.

    ✓ **Role in Soap**: This oil helps create a firm soap with a lot of lather. However, it can be drying if used in large quantities, so it's often balanced with other oils.

3. **Castor Oil**:

    ✓ **Properties**: Castor oil is thick and sticky, which might not seem appealing, but it's fantastic for soap making. It acts as a humectant, drawing moisture to the skin.

- ✓ **Role in Soap**: Castor oil boosts lather and gives the soap a silky, luxurious feel. It's typically used in smaller amounts due to its potent nature.

4. **Jojoba Oil**:

- ✓ **Properties**: Jojoba oil is actually a liquid wax that closely resembles the skin's natural sebum. It's excellent for moisturizing and conditioning the skin.

- ✓ **Role in Soap**: Jojoba oil adds a nourishing touch to soap and is particularly beneficial in liquid soaps intended for facial use or sensitive skin.

5. **Shea Butter**:

- ✓ **Properties**: Shea butter is incredibly moisturizing and rich in vitamins A and E. It helps soothe and protect the skin.

- ✓ **Role in Soap**: While not a liquid oil, shea butter can be melted and combined with other oils to enhance the moisturizing properties of your soap.

Alkali (Potassium Hydroxide)

Potassium hydroxide (KOH) is a crucial ingredient in the soap-making process. It's the alkali that reacts with the oils and fats to create soap through a process called saponification.

- ✓ **Properties**: Potassium hydroxide is a strong base and needs to be handled with care. It's different from sodium hydroxide (NaOH), which is used for making solid bar soaps.

- ✓ **Role in Soap**: KOH breaks down the fats and oils, transforming them into soap and glycerin. This reaction not only cleanses but also helps to maintain the soap in a liquid state.

Distilled Water

Water is essential in soap making for dissolving the potassium hydroxide and diluting the soap paste.

- ✓ **Properties**: Distilled water is free from impurities and minerals that can interfere with the saponification process.

✓ **Role in Soap**: It helps to evenly distribute the KOH throughout the oils and later dilutes the thick soap paste into a pourable liquid soap. Using distilled water ensures that your soap remains clear and free from any unwanted residues.

Additives (Optional but Beneficial)

Additives allow you to personalize your soap, enhancing its scent, color, and beneficial properties. Here are some popular choices:

1. **Fragrance Oils and Essential Oils**:

   ✓ **Properties**: These oils add delightful scents to your soap. Essential oils also come with various therapeutic benefits.

   ✓ **Role in Soap**: They make the soap more pleasant to use and can provide aromatherapy benefits. Popular choices include lavender, peppermint, eucalyptus, and citrus oils.

2. **Colorants**:

- ✓ **Properties**: Colorants can be natural or synthetic. Natural options include mica powders, clays, and herbal powders.

- ✓ **Role in Soap**: They add visual appeal to your soap, making it more attractive and fun to use.

3. **Aloe Vera**:

- ✓ **Properties**: Aloe vera is soothing and healing, known for its ability to calm irritated skin.

- ✓ **Role in Soap**: It enhances the moisturizing properties and adds a soothing quality, making the soap ideal for sensitive or sun-exposed skin.

4. **Vitamin E**:

- ✓ **Properties**: Vitamin E is a powerful antioxidant that helps to nourish and protect the skin.

✓ **Role in Soap**: It extends the shelf life of the soap by preventing the oils from becoming rancid and provides additional skin benefits.

Understanding these essential ingredients is the first step toward successful soap making. Each ingredient brings its own unique properties and benefits to the table, allowing you to create a customized product that meets your specific needs and preferences. By carefully selecting and combining these ingredients, you can craft a liquid soap that is not only effective at cleaning but also gentle and beneficial for your skin. So, gather your ingredients, put on your safety gear, and get ready to dive into the wonderful world of liquid soap making!

2.1.1. Oils and Fats

Oils and fats are the cornerstone of any soap recipe. They are the primary ingredients that determine the characteristics of the final soap product, including its lather, moisturizing properties, hardness, and overall feel. Each type of oil and fat brings unique qualities to the soap, making it important to understand their individual properties and how they interact in the soap-making process. Let's explore some of the most commonly used oils and fats in liquid soap making.

Olive Oil

Properties: Olive oil is renowned for its gentle, moisturizing qualities. It is rich in vitamins A and E, antioxidants, and essential fatty acids, making it incredibly nourishing for the skin.

Role in Soap: Olive oil produces a mild, creamy lather that is less bubbly but more conditioning. It's ideal for sensitive skin and contributes to the soap's overall moisturizing properties. Olive oil-based soaps are often referred to as "Castile soaps," a nod to their origin in the Castile region of Spain, where they were traditionally made from pure olive oil.

Coconut Oil

Properties: Coconut oil is a powerhouse in soap making, known for its ability to create a rich, bubbly lather. It is also noted for its cleansing properties and is often used in higher percentages in soaps meant for oily or acne-prone skin. Coconut oil contains medium-chain fatty acids like lauric acid, which have natural antibacterial and antifungal properties.

HOMEMADE LIQUID SOAP MAKING

Role in Soap: Coconut oil contributes to a soap that lathers well and cleans effectively. However, it can be drying if used in large amounts, so it's typically balanced with more conditioning oils. In liquid soap making, coconut oil helps to create a soap that rinses cleanly, leaving the skin feeling refreshed.

Castor Oil

Properties: Castor oil is thick, viscous, and acts as a humectant, meaning it attracts and retains moisture. It is rich in ricinoleic acid, which gives it a unique ability to provide a rich, creamy lather and contribute to the soap's conditioning properties.

Role in Soap: Castor oil is often used in smaller amounts (typically around 5-10% of the total oils) because of its potent properties. It enhances lather stability and adds a silky feel to the soap, making it a key ingredient in liquid soaps that aim for a luxurious texture.

Jojoba Oil

Properties: Jojoba oil is technically a liquid wax ester, which closely resembles the natural sebum produced by human skin. It is non-comedogenic (won't clog pores) and has excellent moisturizing and conditioning properties.

Role in Soap: Jojoba oil adds a nourishing touch to liquid soaps, making them especially suitable for facial cleansers or products intended for sensitive skin. It also helps to extend the shelf life of the soap due to its stable nature.

Shea Butter

Properties: Shea butter is derived from the nuts of the African shea tree. It is packed with vitamins A and E, essential fatty acids, and other nutrients that are incredibly beneficial for the skin. Shea butter is known for its deep moisturizing and healing properties.

Role in Soap: Although not a liquid oil, shea butter can be melted and combined with other oils to enhance the moisturizing properties of your soap. It adds a creamy texture and contributes to the soap's conditioning qualities, making it a great addition to liquid soaps designed for dry or mature skin.

Sunflower Oil

Properties: Sunflower oil is high in vitamins A, D, and E, and is rich in oleic acid. It is light, non-greasy, and easily absorbed by the skin, making it an excellent choice for soap making.

HOMEMADE LIQUID SOAP MAKING

Role in Soap: Sunflower oil adds moisturizing properties and creates a stable lather. It's particularly good for sensitive skin and helps to balance the overall composition of the soap, ensuring it's not too heavy or too drying.

Avocado Oil

Properties: Avocado oil is deeply penetrating and rich in vitamins A, D, and E. It is known for its regenerative and moisturizing properties, making it ideal for mature, dry, or sensitive skin.

Role in Soap: Avocado oil enhances the conditioning properties of the soap, providing a silky, nourishing feel. It's often used in combination with other oils to create a well-rounded liquid soap that is both cleansing and moisturizing.

Almond Oil

Properties: Almond oil is gentle and moisturizing, rich in vitamins E and K. It is known for its ability to soften and smooth the skin.

Role in Soap: Almond oil adds a luxurious feel to liquid soap, making it gentle and suitable for all skin types, including sensitive skin. It helps to create a balanced soap that cleanses without stripping the skin of its natural oils.

Choosing the right combination of oils and fats is crucial in crafting high-quality liquid soap. Each oil and fat contributes unique properties that affect the soap's performance and feel. By understanding these properties, you can tailor your soap recipes to achieve the desired balance of lather, moisturization, and cleansing power. Whether you prefer a rich, bubbly lather or a creamy, moisturizing wash, the right blend of oils and fats will help you create the perfect liquid soap for your needs.

2.1.2. Lye (Potassium Hydroxide)

When it comes to making liquid soap, lye (specifically potassium hydroxide, or KOH) is an indispensable ingredient. This strong alkali is what transforms oils and fats into soap through a chemical process called saponification. Understanding the role of potassium hydroxide, how to handle it safely, and its specific use in liquid soap making is essential for any aspiring soap maker.

The Role of Potassium Hydroxide in Soap Making

Chemical Reaction: Potassium hydroxide is a caustic alkali that reacts with fats and oils to produce soap and glycerin. This reaction, known as saponification, breaks down the triglycerides in fats and oils into fatty acid salts (the soap) and glycerol (glycerin).

Difference from Sodium Hydroxide: While sodium hydroxide (NaOH) is used for making solid bar soap, potassium hydroxide is preferred for liquid soap. This is because KOH produces a soap that is softer and more soluble in water, resulting in a liquid or gel-like consistency rather than a solid bar.

Properties of Potassium Hydroxide

Strong Alkali: Potassium hydroxide is highly alkaline, with a pH of around 14 in its pure form. This strong alkalinity is necessary for breaking down the fats and oils during the saponification process.

Hygroscopic Nature: Potassium hydroxide is hygroscopic, meaning it absorbs moisture from the air. This property requires it to be stored in airtight containers to prevent it from becoming clumpy or reacting prematurely with moisture in the air.

HOMEMADE LIQUID SOAP MAKING

Handling and Safety: Due to its caustic nature, potassium hydroxide must be handled with care. Proper safety gear, including gloves, goggles, and an apron, is essential to protect your skin and eyes from potential burns or irritation.

Using Potassium Hydroxide in Liquid Soap Making

Preparing the Lye Solution: To prepare the lye solution, you'll need to dissolve potassium hydroxide in water. This step generates heat and releases fumes, so it should always be done in a well-ventilated area. Remember to add the lye to the water, never the other way around, to prevent splashing and a possible exothermic reaction.

1. **Measuring**: Accurate measurement is crucial. Use a digital scale to weigh the potassium hydroxide and distilled water precisely according to your recipe. Soap making is a precise science, and even small deviations can affect the final product.

2. **Mixing**: Slowly add the potassium hydroxide to the distilled water while stirring gently. The solution will heat up and produce fumes, so it's important to do this step carefully. Once the lye is fully dissolved, allow the solution to cool to the desired temperature before combining it with the oils.

HOMEMADE LIQUID SOAP MAKING

Safety Precautions

1. **Protective Gear**: Always wear gloves, goggles, and an apron when handling potassium hydroxide. This will protect your skin and eyes from potential splashes and spills.

2. **Ventilation**: Work in a well-ventilated area or use a fume hood to avoid inhaling the fumes produced when mixing the lye solution.

3. **Emergency Measures**: Keep vinegar nearby to neutralize any lye that may come into contact with your skin. Rinse the affected area thoroughly with water and seek medical attention if necessary.

4. **Storage**: Store potassium hydroxide in a cool, dry place in a tightly sealed container. This will prevent it from absorbing moisture from the air and maintain its effectiveness for soap making.

Common Concerns and Misconceptions

Lye in Finished Soap: A common concern among beginners is the presence of lye in the finished soap. It's important to understand that when properly made, no lye remains in the finished product. The saponification process completely transforms the lye and oils into soap and glycerin, leaving no residual lye.

Environmental Impact: Potassium hydroxide is biodegradable, and soaps made with it are generally environmentally friendly. However, it's important to use and dispose of all chemicals responsibly.

Potassium hydroxide is a critical ingredient in liquid soap making, enabling the transformation of oils and fats into soap through the process of saponification. While it requires careful handling due to its caustic nature, understanding its properties and role in soap making ensures a safe and successful soap-making experience. By respecting the power of potassium hydroxide and following proper safety protocols, you can create high-quality liquid soaps that are effective, gentle, and tailored to your needs.

2.1.3. Water

Water is an essential component in the process of making liquid soap. It serves multiple crucial roles, from dissolving lye to diluting the soap paste. Using the right type of water and understanding its functions in soap making are key to achieving a successful and high-quality product.

The Role of Water in Soap Making

Dissolving Lye: Water is used to dissolve potassium hydroxide (KOH), creating a lye solution necessary for the saponification process. This solution, when mixed with oils, initiates the chemical reaction that turns fats into soap.

Diluting Soap Paste: After the saponification process, the soap paste needs to be diluted to achieve the desired liquid consistency. Water is added gradually to break down the thick soap paste into a smooth, pourable liquid soap.

Balancing Consistency: The amount of water used in the dilution process determines the thickness of the final soap. By adjusting the water content, you can create anything from a thick, gel-like soap to a thin, watery consistency.

Choosing the Right Type of Water

Distilled Water: The best choice for soap making is distilled water. Distilled water is free from impurities, minerals, and contaminants that can interfere with the saponification process and affect the clarity and quality of the final soap product.

- ✓ **Why Distilled Water?**: Tap water can contain minerals, chlorine, and other impurities that may react with the soap ingredients, leading to undesirable results such as cloudiness, reduced lather, or even soap scum. Using distilled water ensures a purer, more predictable reaction and a clearer final product.

Other Types of Water: While distilled water is preferred, other types of water can be used in a pinch, though they may not yield as consistent results.

- ✓ **Filtered Water**: If distilled water is not available, filtered water is a better alternative than tap water. It removes some impurities, but not as effectively as distilled water.

- ✓ **Rainwater**: In some cases, rainwater can be used if it is collected and stored properly to ensure it is free from contaminants. However, it is less predictable than distilled water.

Handling and Measuring Water

Accurate Measurement: Precise measurement of water is crucial in soap making. Using too little water can result in an overly thick or unmanageable soap paste, while too much water can make the soap too thin and runny.

- ✓ **Digital Scale**: Use a digital scale to measure water accurately. Soap making is a precise science, and even small deviations in water content can affect the final product.

Safety Precautions: When mixing water with potassium hydroxide, always add the lye to the water, never the other way around. This prevents a violent exothermic reaction that can cause the solution to splash and potentially cause burns.

Water in the Dilution Process

Gradual Addition: When diluting the soap paste, add water gradually. This allows you to control the consistency of the soap more effectively and prevents the paste from becoming too thin too quickly.

Heating the Water: Using warm water during the dilution process can help the soap paste dissolve more easily and speed up the process. However, avoid using boiling water as it can cause the soap to foam excessively.

Resting Period: After adding water to the soap paste, allow the mixture to rest. This resting period helps the soap paste fully absorb the water and reach a consistent texture. Stir occasionally to check the consistency and add more water if necessary.

Troubleshooting Water Issues

Cloudy Soap: If your soap becomes cloudy after dilution, it may be due to impurities in the water or too much water. Using distilled water and measuring accurately can help prevent this issue.

Separation: If the soap and water separate after dilution, it could be a sign of improper saponification or incorrect measurements. Re-blending the mixture and ensuring accurate measurements in future batches can help resolve this problem.

Water is a vital ingredient in liquid soap making, playing multiple roles from dissolving lye to diluting the soap paste. Using distilled water ensures a pure, high-quality final product, free from impurities that can affect the soap's performance and appearance. Accurate measurement and careful handling of water are essential to achieving the desired consistency and clarity in your liquid soap. By understanding the importance of water and how to use it effectively, you can create a successful and satisfying soap-making experience.

2.1.4. Additives (Fragrances, Colorants, etc.)

Additives play a significant role in enhancing the appeal and functionality of liquid soap. They allow soap makers to personalize their creations, adding scents, colors, and additional beneficial properties to the final product. Understanding how to incorporate additives into your liquid soap recipes can elevate both the aesthetic and functional aspects of your soap-making endeavors.

Fragrances

Types of Fragrances:

1. **Fragrance Oils**: These are synthetic or blended oils specifically formulated for soap making. They offer a wide range of scents, from floral and fruity to exotic and spicy.

2. **Essential Oils**: Derived from natural plant sources, essential oils provide both scent and therapeutic benefits. Popular choices include lavender for relaxation, peppermint for freshness, and citrus oils for invigoration.

Incorporating Fragrances:

1. **Usage Rates**: Fragrance oils are typically used at a rate of 1-3% of the total soap recipe, depending on the desired strength of the scent. Essential oils may require slightly higher concentrations due to their potency.

2. **Timing**: Fragrances should be added to the soap mixture after saponification, during the dilution phase. This ensures that the scent is retained without being altered by the chemical reaction.

Considerations:

✓ **Skin Sensitivity**: Some fragrances, particularly synthetic fragrance oils, may cause skin irritation or allergic reactions in sensitive individuals. Always perform a patch test and consider your target audience when selecting fragrances.

Colorants

HOMEMADE LIQUID SOAP MAKING

Types of Colorants:

1. **Mica Powders**: These are mineral-based powders that provide shimmer and color to soap. They come in a wide range of colors and are stable in soap formulations.

2. **Natural Colorants**: Examples include clays (e.g., French green clay, kaolin clay), herbal powders (e.g., turmeric, spirulina), and botanical extracts. These additives offer natural hues and may provide additional skin benefits.

3. **Synthetic Colorants**: Liquid soap dyes or water-soluble dyes are synthetic options that offer vibrant colors. They are often used in smaller quantities due to their concentrated nature.

Incorporating Colorants:

1. **Preparation**: Mix colorants with a small amount of liquid soap base or glycerin before adding them to the main batch. This ensures even distribution and prevents clumping.

2. **Amount**: Start with a small amount of colorant and gradually increase until the desired hue is achieved.

Remember that the color may intensify as the soap cures.

Considerations:

- ✓ **Staining**: Some colorants, especially natural options like turmeric or spirulina, may stain fabrics or surfaces. Take precautions to avoid spills and thoroughly clean equipment after use.

- ✓ **Fade Resistance**: Natural colorants may fade over time, especially when exposed to light and air. Store colored soaps in opaque or tinted containers to preserve their vibrancy.

Additional Additives

Glycerin: Glycerin is a natural byproduct of the saponification process and acts as a humectant, attracting moisture to the skin. It enhances the soap's moisturizing properties and can be added in small amounts to liquid soap formulations.

Botanicals and Exfoliants: Dried herbs, flower petals, oatmeal, or coffee grounds can be incorporated into liquid soap for visual appeal and gentle exfoliation. Ensure that these additives are finely ground and suitable for use on the skin.

Specialty Ingredients: Consider adding ingredients like aloe vera gel, silk peptides, or honey for their skin-soothing and conditioning properties. These additives can elevate the functionality of your liquid soap, making it more appealing to consumers seeking specific benefits.

Additives offer endless possibilities for customizing and enhancing liquid soap recipes. Whether you're aiming to create a visually stunning product, add therapeutic scents, or incorporate additional skincare benefits, understanding the characteristics and proper usage of additives is crucial. By experimenting with different fragrances, colorants, and specialty ingredients, you can create unique liquid soaps that cater to diverse preferences and needs. Always prioritize safety, accuracy in measurement, and quality sourcing when selecting and incorporating additives into your soap-making process.

2.2. Necessary Equipment

To successfully craft liquid soap at home, having the right equipment is essential. Proper tools not only facilitate the soap-making process but also ensure safety and consistency in your final product. Here's a comprehensive list of the necessary equipment you'll need:

1. Heat-Resistant Containers

Purpose: Heat-resistant containers are used for mixing and heating ingredients, especially when preparing the lye solution and diluting the soap paste.

Types:

- ✓ **Stainless Steel**: Durable and easy to clean, stainless steel containers are ideal for handling caustic substances like potassium hydroxide.

- ✓ **Heat-Resistant Plastic**: Some plastic containers are specifically designed to withstand heat and are suitable for mixing lye solutions. Ensure they are labeled as heat-resistant and safe for use with lye.

2. Digital Scale

Purpose: Accurate measurement of ingredients is crucial in soap making to ensure consistency and predictable results.

Features:

- ✓ **Precision**: Choose a digital scale that measures in grams or ounces with high accuracy. This allows you to weigh oils, potassium hydroxide (KOH), and other additives precisely according to your soap recipe.

3. Stick Blender

Purpose: A stick blender, also known as an immersion blender, is used to emulsify and blend the oils, potassium hydroxide, and water during the soap-making process.

Features:

- ✓ **Stainless Steel Shaft**: Opt for a stick blender with a stainless steel shaft, as it is resistant to corrosion from caustic materials like KOH.

- ✓ **Variable Speeds**: Variable speed settings provide control over the blending process, ensuring thorough emulsification and mixing of ingredients.

4. Thermometer

Purpose: Monitoring temperatures during the soap-making process is critical for safely handling lye and achieving the correct consistency of soap mixtures.

Types:

✓ **Digital Thermometer**: Digital thermometers provide quick and accurate temperature readings, making them ideal for monitoring lye solution temperatures and ensuring they are within safe ranges.

5. Safety Gear

Purpose: Safety gear protects you from potential hazards associated with handling lye and other caustic materials.

Essential Items:

✓ **Rubber Gloves**: Chemical-resistant gloves protect your hands from lye and caustic solutions.

✓ **Safety Goggles**: Goggles shield your eyes from splashes and fumes when mixing lye and water.

✓ **Apron**: An apron helps protect your clothing from spills and splashes during the soap-making process.

6. pH Strips or pH Meter

Purpose: pH testing is crucial to ensure that the soap mixture has fully saponified and is safe for use.

Types:

- ✓ **pH Strips**: pH strips provide a quick and convenient method to check the acidity or alkalinity of your soap mixture.

- ✓ **pH Meter**: A pH meter offers precise pH readings and is ideal for more accurate testing of soap formulations.

7. Mixing Spoons and Spatulas

Purpose: Mixing spoons and spatulas are used for stirring and combining ingredients during different stages of soap making.

Features:

- ✓ **Non-Reactive Materials**: Choose spoons and spatulas made from non-reactive materials such as stainless steel or silicone to avoid chemical reactions with lye.

8. Measuring Cups and Pouring Containers

Purpose: Measuring cups and pouring containers are essential for accurately measuring and dispensing liquid ingredients like oils, water, and fragrance.

Types:

- ✓ **Glass Measuring Cups**: Glass measuring cups are durable and heat-resistant, making them suitable for measuring and pouring hot liquids.

- ✓ **Plastic Pouring Containers**: Plastic containers with spouts facilitate controlled pouring of soap mixtures into molds or bottles.

9. Soap Mold or Storage Containers

Purpose: Soap molds or storage containers are used to shape and store your liquid soap as it cures and solidifies.

Options:

- ✓ **Silicone Soap Molds**: Flexible silicone molds are ideal for liquid soap making, as they allow for easy removal of the soap once it has cured.

- ✓ **Storage Bottles**: Use storage bottles with dispensing pumps for storing and using liquid soap. Choose containers made from materials that are compatible with liquid soap ingredients to prevent reactions or deterioration.

10. Labels and Packaging Materials

Purpose: Labels and packaging materials are used for identifying and storing your finished liquid soap products.

Items:

- ✓ **Waterproof Labels**: Waterproof labels ensure that labels remain intact and legible, even when exposed to water or moisture.

- ✓ **Storage Containers**: Use air-tight containers or bottles to store liquid soap, protecting it from contaminants and maintaining its quality.

Having the right equipment is essential for successful liquid soap making at home. Each tool and safety gear item plays a crucial role in ensuring the accurate measurement, safe handling, and effective mixing of ingredients. By investing in quality equipment and following proper soap-making procedures, you can create high-quality liquid soaps tailored to your preferences and needs. Always prioritize safety and accuracy to achieve consistent and satisfying results in your soap-making endeavors.

2.2.1. Safety Gear

Safety gear is essential when making liquid soap, especially when handling caustic materials like potassium hydroxide (KOH). Protecting yourself from potential hazards ensures a safe and enjoyable soap-making experience. Here are the essential safety gear items you'll need:

HOMEMADE LIQUID SOAP MAKING

1. Rubber Gloves

Purpose: Rubber gloves protect your hands from direct contact with potassium hydroxide and other caustic substances used in soap making.

Features:

- ✓ **Chemical-Resistant**: Choose gloves specifically designed to resist chemicals and alkalis like KOH.

- ✓ **Comfortable Fit**: Ensure gloves fit snugly to provide maximum protection without compromising dexterity.

2. Safety Goggles

Purpose: Safety goggles shield your eyes from splashes, fumes, and accidental spills during the soap-making process.

Features:

- ✓ **Full Coverage**: Opt for goggles that provide a secure fit and cover your eyes completely to prevent any exposure to lye or other chemicals.

- ✓ **Anti-Fog Coating**: Anti-fog goggles are beneficial to maintain clear vision, especially when working in humid conditions.

3. Apron

Purpose: An apron protects your clothing from spills and splashes of lye solution and soap ingredients.

Features:

- ✓ **Waterproof or Chemical-Resistant**: Choose an apron made from materials that can withstand contact with liquids and chemicals.

- ✓ **Coverage**: Ensure the apron covers your torso and legs adequately to protect against accidental spills.

4. Face Mask or Respirator

Purpose: A face mask or respirator protects your respiratory system from inhaling fumes and vapors during the soap-making process.

Types:

- ✓ **Respirator**: Use a respirator with cartridges designed for protection against chemical vapors if working in a poorly ventilated area or handling large quantities of potassium hydroxide.

✓ **Face Mask**: A face mask may suffice for general use if working in a well-ventilated space. Choose masks rated for chemical fume protection if necessary.

5. Closed-Toe Shoes

Purpose: Closed-toe shoes provide protection for your feet against spills and accidental splashes of lye solution or soap mixtures.

Features:

✓ **Durable Construction**: Choose shoes made from durable materials that offer protection and comfort during prolonged periods of standing and mixing.

6. Long-Sleeved Clothing

Purpose: Long-sleeved clothing provides an additional layer of protection against accidental spills and splashes during soap making.

Features:

✓ **Comfortable Fabric**: Wear comfortable clothing made from natural fibers like cotton to minimize heat retention and discomfort while working.

Additional Tips for Safety

- ✓ **Ventilation**: Work in a well-ventilated area or use a fume hood to minimize exposure to vapors and fumes from lye and other chemicals.

- ✓ **Emergency Preparedness**: Keep a bottle of vinegar nearby to neutralize any spills or splashes of lye on skin. Rinse affected areas with water immediately and seek medical attention if irritation occurs.

- ✓ **Storage**: Store potassium hydroxide and other chemicals in tightly sealed containers in a cool, dry place away from children and pets.

Safety gear is essential for protecting yourself from potential hazards when making liquid soap. By wearing rubber gloves, safety goggles, an apron, and appropriate respiratory protection, you can minimize risks and ensure a safe soap-making experience. Always prioritize safety protocols, proper ventilation, and emergency preparedness to handle any unexpected situations during the soap-making process.

2.2.2. Mixing and Heating Tools

Having the right mixing and heating tools is crucial for effectively and safely making liquid soap at home. These tools facilitate the blending of ingredients, ensure proper temperature control, and contribute to the overall quality of your soap. Here are the essential mixing and heating tools you'll need:

1. Heat-Resistant Containers

Purpose: Heat-resistant containers are used for mixing and heating ingredients, especially when preparing the lye solution and diluting the soap paste.

Types:

- ✓ **Stainless Steel Containers**: Durable and easy to clean, stainless steel containers are ideal for handling hot liquids and caustic substances like potassium hydroxide (KOH).

- ✓ **Heat-Resistant Plastic Containers**: Some plastic containers are designed to withstand heat and are suitable for mixing lye solutions. Ensure they are labeled as heat-resistant and safe for use with lye.

2. Stick Blender (Immersion Blender)

Purpose: A stick blender is essential for emulsifying and blending the oils, potassium hydroxide, and water during the soap-making process.

Features:

- ✓ **Stainless Steel Shaft**: Opt for a stick blender with a stainless steel shaft, as it is resistant to corrosion from caustic materials like KOH.

- ✓ **Variable Speeds**: Variable speed settings provide control over the blending process, ensuring thorough emulsification and mixing of ingredients.

3. Digital Scale

Purpose: Accurate measurement of ingredients is crucial in soap making to ensure consistency and predictable results.

Features:

- ✓ **Precision**: Choose a digital scale that measures in grams or ounces with high accuracy. This allows you to weigh oils, potassium hydroxide (KOH), and other additives precisely according to your soap recipe.

4. Thermometer

Purpose: Monitoring temperatures during the soap-making process is critical for safely handling lye and achieving the correct consistency of soap mixtures.

Types:

- ✓ **Digital Thermometer**: Digital thermometers provide quick and accurate temperature readings, making them ideal for monitoring lye solution temperatures and ensuring they are within safe ranges.

5. Mixing Spoons and Spatulas

Purpose: Mixing spoons and spatulas are used for stirring and combining ingredients during different stages of soap making.

Features:

- ✓ **Non-Reactive Materials**: Choose spoons and spatulas made from non-reactive materials such as stainless steel or silicone to avoid chemical reactions with lye.

6. Double Boiler or Water Bath Setup

Purpose: A double boiler or water bath setup is used for gently heating and melting solid oils or butter, ensuring they are fully incorporated into the soap mixture.

Features:

- ✓ **Safety**: Prevents direct heat exposure to oils, minimizing the risk of scorching or overheating.

- ✓ **Stability**: Provides a stable and controlled environment for heating ingredients without direct contact with an open flame or burner.

7. pH Strips or pH Meter

Purpose: pH testing is crucial to ensure that the soap mixture has fully saponified and is safe for use.

Types:

- ✓ **pH Strips**: pH strips provide a quick and convenient method to check the acidity or alkalinity of your soap mixture.

- ✓ **pH Meter**: A pH meter offers precise pH readings and is ideal for more accurate testing of soap formulations.

8. Containers for Dilution and Storage

Purpose: Use containers with spouts for diluting the soap paste and pouring the finished liquid soap into storage bottles or molds.

Types:

- ✓ **Glass Measuring Cups**: Glass measuring cups are durable and heat-resistant, making them suitable for measuring and pouring hot liquids.

- ✓ **Plastic Pouring Containers**: Plastic containers with spouts facilitate controlled pouring of soap mixtures into molds or bottles.

Mixing and heating tools are essential for successful liquid soap making at home. Each tool serves a specific purpose, from accurately measuring ingredients to blending them to the right consistency and ensuring safe handling of lye and other components. By investing in quality equipment and following proper soap-making procedures, you can create high-quality liquid soaps tailored to your preferences and needs. Always prioritize safety, accuracy in measurement, and quality sourcing when selecting and using mixing and heating tools in your soap-making process.

2.2.3. Measuring and Storage Containers

Having appropriate measuring and storage containers is crucial for accurately portioning ingredients and storing your liquid soap safely. These containers ensure precise measurements during the soap-making process and provide convenient storage solutions for your finished products. Here's what you'll need:

1. Measuring Cups and Spoons

Purpose: Measuring cups and spoons are essential for accurately measuring liquid and dry ingredients used in your soap recipes.

Features:

- ✓ **Variety of Sizes**: Have measuring cups and spoons in various sizes (e.g., 1 cup, ½ cup, 1 tablespoon) to accommodate different ingredient quantities.

- ✓ **Material**: Choose cups and spoons made from durable materials such as stainless steel or heat-resistant plastic for ease of cleaning and durability.

2. Digital Scale

Purpose: A digital scale provides precise measurements of oils, potassium hydroxide (KOH), and other ingredients by weight, ensuring consistency in your soap recipes.

Features:

- ✓ **Accuracy**: Opt for a digital scale that measures in grams or ounces with high accuracy, especially when working with small amounts of additives and fragrances.

- ✓ **Tare Function**: The tare function allows you to zero out the weight of the container, making it easier to measure ingredients directly into mixing containers without calculations.

3. Graduated Pitchers or Containers with Volume Markings

Purpose: Graduated pitchers and containers with volume markings are used for measuring and mixing larger quantities of liquid ingredients like water and diluted soap paste.

Features:

- ✓ **Clear Measurement Markings**: Ensure containers have clear, easy-to-read volume markings to accurately measure liquids and monitor levels during mixing.

- ✓ **Material**: Choose containers made from sturdy materials like plastic or glass that can withstand the heat and chemical exposure typical in soap making.

4. Storage Bottles or Containers

Purpose: Storage bottles or containers are used to store and dispense your finished liquid soap.

Features:

- ✓ **Material Compatibility**: Select bottles or containers made from materials compatible with liquid soap ingredients to prevent reactions or deterioration.

- ✓ **Dispensing Options**: Choose containers with dispensing pumps for convenient use in bathrooms or kitchens. Alternatively, use jars with secure lids for storing larger batches.

5. Mixing Bowls and Mixing Containers

Purpose: Mixing bowls and containers are used for combining and blending soap ingredients before pouring them into molds or storage bottles.

Features:

- ✓ **Non-Reactive Materials**: Use bowls and containers made from non-reactive materials such as stainless steel, glass, or heat-resistant plastic to avoid chemical interactions with soap ingredients.

- ✓ **Size Variability**: Have a range of sizes available to accommodate different batch sizes and ensure thorough mixing without overflow.

6. Funnel

Purpose: A funnel facilitates pouring liquid soap into smaller bottles or molds without spills or mess.

Features:

- ✓ **Wide Opening**: Choose a funnel with a wide opening to accommodate thicker soap mixtures without clogging.

✓ **Material**: Opt for funnels made from stainless steel or food-grade plastic for durability and ease of cleaning.

7. Labels

Purpose: Labels are used to identify and provide information about your liquid soap products.

Features:

✓ **Waterproof**: Use waterproof labels or stickers to ensure they remain intact and legible, even when exposed to moisture.

✓ **Information**: Include details such as the soap name, ingredients, date of production, and any usage instructions or precautions.

8. Storage Containers for Ingredients

Purpose: Store bulk quantities of ingredients like oils, potassium hydroxide (KOH), fragrance oils, and colorants in tightly sealed containers to maintain freshness and quality.

Features:

✓ **Air-Tight Seal**: Containers should have air-tight seals to prevent oxidation and maintain the potency of oils and additives.

✓ **Dark or Opaque Containers**: Use dark or opaque containers to protect light-sensitive ingredients like essential oils and natural colorants from degradation.

Measuring and storage containers are essential tools for successful liquid soap making. They ensure accurate ingredient measurements, facilitate efficient mixing and blending, and provide secure storage for your finished products. By using durable, non-reactive materials and organizing your workspace with the right containers, you can streamline your soap-making process and create high-quality liquid soaps tailored to your preferences and needs. Always label containers properly and store ingredients in optimal conditions to maintain their effectiveness and prolong shelf life.

CHAPTER THREE

SAFETY PRECAUTIONS

3.1. Handling Lye Safely

When making liquid soap, handling lye (potassium hydroxide) requires careful attention and adherence to safety protocols. Lye is a caustic substance that can cause severe burns and irritation if mishandled. By following these safety precautions, you can ensure a safe and successful soap-making experience:

Understanding Lye

Caution: Lye, also known as potassium hydroxide (KOH), is a highly alkaline substance used in soap making to saponify oils and create soap. It can cause severe burns if it comes into contact with skin, eyes, or mucous membranes.

Safety Gear

1. Rubber Gloves: Always wear chemical-resistant gloves when handling lye to protect your hands from accidental spills or splashes.

2. Safety Goggles: Protect your eyes with safety goggles to shield them from lye splashes or fumes.

3. Long-Sleeved Clothing: Wear long sleeves and pants to minimize skin exposure to lye.

4. Closed-Toe Shoes: Use closed-toe shoes to protect your feet from spills.

Workspace Preparation

5. Well-Ventilated Area: Work in a well-ventilated space to minimize inhalation of lye fumes. Consider using a fume hood if available.

6. Clear Workspace: Ensure your workspace is clean and free of clutter to avoid accidents.

Handling Lye Safely

7. Add Lye to Water: Always add lye to water (never the other way around) to prevent violent splattering. Use cold water and slowly sprinkle lye into it while stirring gently.

8. Mix Outdoors or Under Ventilation: Mix lye solution outdoors or under a ventilation hood to minimize exposure to fumes.

9. Use Heat-Resistant Containers: Use heat-resistant containers (such as stainless steel or heat-resistant plastic) when mixing lye solution. Avoid glass containers, as they can crack due to the heat generated during the mixing process.

Emergency Preparedness

10. Vinegar Solution: Keep a bottle of vinegar nearby. If lye comes into contact with your skin, immediately flush the affected area with vinegar to neutralize the alkali. Rinse thoroughly with water afterward.

11. First Aid Kit: Have a first aid kit accessible with supplies for treating chemical burns, such as burn cream and sterile dressings.

Clean-Up and Storage

12. Clean-Up: Clean all equipment and surfaces that come into contact with lye thoroughly after use. Use plenty of water to rinse away any residue.

13. Storage: Store lye in a secure, dry place, out of reach of children and pets. Keep it tightly sealed in its original container to prevent moisture absorption.

Educational Resources

14. Educate Yourself: Before using lye for soap making, educate yourself on its properties, safe handling procedures, and emergency response protocols.

Handling lye safely is paramount in liquid soap making to prevent accidents and ensure personal safety. By wearing protective gear, working in a well-ventilated area, and following precise mixing procedures, you can minimize risks and enjoy a rewarding soap-making experience. Always prioritize safety and take necessary precautions to protect yourself and others from potential hazards associated with handling lye.

3.2. Personal Protective Equipment

When working with lye and other potentially hazardous materials in liquid soap making, Personal Protective Equipment (PPE) is your first line of defense. Wearing the right PPE ensures your safety, prevents accidents, and allows you to focus on creating high-quality soap. Here's a detailed guide to the essential PPE you should use:

1. Rubber Gloves

Purpose: Rubber gloves protect your hands from lye and other caustic substances, preventing burns and irritation.

Features:

- ✓ **Chemical-Resistant**: Choose gloves specifically designed for chemical resistance. Nitrile or neoprene gloves are ideal as they provide excellent protection against lye.

✓ **Length**: Opt for long gloves that extend up to your forearms to protect more of your skin from splashes.

Usage Tips:

✓ **Inspect Before Use**: Always check gloves for any tears or holes before putting them on.

✓ **Replace Regularly**: Replace gloves if they become worn or damaged during use.

2. Safety Goggles

Purpose: Safety goggles protect your eyes from lye splashes, preventing severe eye damage or blindness.

Features:

✓ **Full Coverage**: Choose goggles that offer complete coverage around your eyes to prevent any lye from reaching them.

✓ **Anti-Fog Coating**: Opt for goggles with an anti-fog coating for clear vision, especially in humid environments.

Usage Tips:

- ✓ **Fit Properly**: Ensure goggles fit snugly to your face without gaps. This prevents lye vapors or droplets from entering.

3. Apron

Purpose: An apron protects your clothing and skin from spills and splashes of lye and soap mixture.

Features:

- ✓ **Material**: Use aprons made from waterproof or chemical-resistant materials, such as PVC or polyurethane.

- ✓ **Coverage**: Choose an apron that covers your torso and extends to your knees to provide maximum protection.

Usage Tips:

- ✓ **Secure Fit**: Ensure the apron has adjustable straps or ties to fit snugly around your waist and neck, preventing accidental exposure.

4. Face Mask or Respirator

Purpose: A face mask or respirator protects your respiratory system from inhaling harmful fumes or dust particles generated during the soap-making process.

Types:

- ✓ **Dust Mask**: For minimal exposure, a dust mask can help filter out large particles.

- ✓ **Respirator**: For higher protection, use a respirator equipped with chemical cartridges designed to filter out toxic fumes.

Features:

- ✓ **Fit and Seal**: Ensure the mask or respirator fits well to create a tight seal around your nose and mouth. This is crucial for effective protection.

Usage Tips:

- ✓ **Replace Filters**: Replace the filters in your respirator regularly according to the manufacturer's instructions.

5. Long-Sleeved Clothing and Pants

Purpose: Long-sleeved clothing and pants protect your skin from lye and potential spills.

Features:

- ✓ **Fabric Choice**: Wear cotton or other natural fibers that are comfortable and provide a barrier against chemical exposure.

- ✓ **Coverage**: Choose clothing that covers your arms and legs completely to minimize skin exposure.

Usage Tips:

- ✓ **Tuck in Clothes**: Tuck your shirt sleeves into your gloves and your pants into your socks or boots to prevent lye from contacting your skin.

6. Closed-Toe Shoes

Purpose: Closed-toe shoes protect your feet from spills and splashes, reducing the risk of burns or irritation.

Features:

✓ **Durable Material**: Choose shoes made from sturdy, chemical-resistant materials. Rubber boots are an excellent option for additional protection.

✓ **Comfort and Fit**: Ensure shoes are comfortable and provide good support for standing and moving around safely in the workspace.

7. Emergency Equipment

Purpose: Having emergency equipment on hand is crucial for quickly addressing accidents or exposure to lye.

Essential Items:

✓ **Vinegar Solution**: Keep a bottle of vinegar nearby to neutralize lye spills on skin. Rinse the affected area thoroughly with water afterward.

✓ **First Aid Kit**: Ensure your first aid kit includes supplies for treating chemical burns, such as burn cream, sterile dressings, and antiseptic wipes.

Usage Tips:

✓ **Know the Location**: Keep all emergency equipment easily accessible and ensure all participants know where it is located.

Personal Protective Equipment (PPE) is indispensable for safe liquid soap making. By wearing the proper gloves, goggles, apron, and other protective gear, you significantly reduce the risk of accidents and injuries. Always prioritize safety, maintain your PPE in good condition, and be prepared to respond quickly to any incidents. With the right precautions, you can enjoy a safe and productive soap-making experience.

3.3. Safe Workspace Setup

Creating a safe workspace is essential for conducting liquid soap making effectively and minimizing potential hazards. A well-organized and properly equipped workspace not only enhances safety but also contributes to the overall success of your soap-making endeavors. Here's how to set up a safe workspace for liquid soap making:

1. Location Selection

Choose a Well-Ventilated Area: Select a workspace that is well-ventilated to ensure proper air circulation. Good ventilation helps disperse any fumes generated during the soap-making process, reducing inhalation risks.

Consider Outdoor or Dedicated Area: If possible, set up your workspace outdoors or in a dedicated area away from living spaces. This minimizes exposure to lye fumes and ensures a controlled environment for handling chemicals.

2. Workspace Preparation

Clear and Clean Surface: Prepare a clean, flat surface for your soap-making activities. Ensure the workspace is free of clutter and other distractions that could lead to accidents.

Cover Surfaces: Protect surfaces with newspaper, plastic sheets, or disposable tablecloths to facilitate easier cleanup of spills and splatters.

3. Access to Utilities

Proximity to Water Source: Position your workspace near a water source for easy access when rinsing equipment, diluting lye, or addressing spills.

Electrical Outlets: Ensure access to electrical outlets for powering equipment such as stick blenders and digital scales. Use ground-fault circuit interrupters (GFCIs) to prevent electrical shocks.

4. Storage and Organization

Secure Storage for Chemicals: Store lye and other chemicals in secure, labeled containers away from children and pets. Ensure containers are tightly sealed to prevent spills and contamination.

Organize Equipment and Supplies: Arrange soap-making equipment, ingredients, and tools in a logical layout. This promotes efficiency during the soap-making process and reduces the risk of accidents caused by reaching over cluttered surfaces.

5. Emergency Preparedness

First Aid Kit: Keep a well-stocked first aid kit readily available in your workspace. Include supplies such as burn cream, sterile dressings, eyewash solution, and emergency contact numbers.

Emergency Response Plan: Develop and communicate an emergency response plan that outlines procedures for handling spills, exposure to lye, or other accidents. Ensure all participants are familiar with the plan and know the location of emergency equipment.

6. Personal Safety Protocols

Use Personal Protective Equipment (PPE): Always wear appropriate PPE, including gloves, safety goggles, apron, and closed-toe shoes, when handling lye and other chemicals. Replace PPE as needed to maintain effectiveness.

Avoid Distractions: Focus solely on the soap-making task at hand to minimize the risk of accidents. Avoid multitasking or engaging in activities that could divert your attention from safe procedures.

7. Cleaning and Maintenance

Regular Equipment Cleaning: Clean and sanitize soap-making equipment regularly to prevent cross-contamination and ensure consistent soap quality.

Inspect and Maintain Tools: Regularly inspect tools and equipment for signs of wear or damage. Replace worn-out or defective items promptly to maintain safe working conditions.

A safe workspace setup is essential for successful and hazard-free liquid soap making. By choosing a well-ventilated location, organizing your workspace efficiently, and prioritizing safety protocols, you can minimize risks and enjoy a productive soap-making experience. Always adhere to safe handling practices, maintain your equipment and supplies, and be prepared to respond to emergencies effectively. With a safe workspace, you can create high-quality liquid soaps confidently and safely.

CHAPTER FOUR

THE LIQUID SOAP MAKING PROCESS

4.1. Preparing the Lye Solution

Preparing the lye solution is a critical step in liquid soap making that requires careful handling and precise measurements to ensure safety and effective saponification. Lye, also known as sodium hydroxide (for bar soap) or potassium hydroxide (for liquid soap), is a necessary chemical component that reacts with oils to form soap.

1. Safety Precautions

- ✓ **Protective Gear**: Before starting, ensure you have protective gear including safety goggles, gloves, and a long-sleeved shirt to shield skin from potential splashes or spills.

- ✓ **Ventilation**: Work in a well-ventilated area to avoid inhaling fumes emitted during the lye mixing process.

HOMEMADE LIQUID SOAP MAKING

2. Ingredients and Equipment

- ✓ **Lye (Potassium Hydroxide)**: Purchase high-quality potassium hydroxide flakes or pellets suitable for soap making.

- ✓ **Distilled Water**: Use distilled water, as it ensures purity and avoids impurities that may interfere with the soap-making process.

3. Measuring and Mixing

- ✓ **Measurements**: Use a digital scale to measure the precise amount of potassium hydroxide required based on your soap recipe. Always refer to a reliable soap-making calculator for accurate proportions.

- ✓ **Mixing Container**: Select a heat-resistant container, such as stainless steel or tempered glass, for mixing the lye solution.

4. Procedure

- ✓ **Safety First**: Put on your protective gear. Start by adding distilled water to your mixing container. Avoid using metal containers or utensils, as lye reacts with metal.

- ✓ **Lye Addition**: Carefully add the potassium hydroxide to the water, not the other way around, to prevent a violent reaction. Stir gently and continuously using a non-reactive spoon until the lye is fully dissolved.

- ✓ **Heat Source**: If necessary according to your recipe, gently heat the mixture using a water bath or indirect heat until the lye is completely dissolved and the solution becomes clear. Do not heat directly on a stovetop or open flame to avoid overheating or splattering.

5. Cooling and Safety Checks

- ✓ **Cooling**: Allow the lye solution to cool naturally to room temperature before using it in the soap-making process. Do not rush this step to prevent accidental splashes or spills.

- ✓ **Safety Check**: Test the temperature of the lye solution with a thermometer to ensure it has cooled adequately for safe handling and mixing with oils.

6. Storage and Handling

- ✓ **Secure Storage**: Once cooled, store the lye solution in a labeled, tightly sealed container away from children and pets. Keep it in a cool, dry place to maintain its effectiveness.

7. Handling Spills or Accidents

✓ **Neutralization**: In case of spills, immediately neutralize with vinegar or citric acid solution. Rinse affected areas with plenty of water to mitigate any potential skin or surface damage.

8. Final Considerations

✓ **Accuracy**: Always double-check your measurements and calculations when preparing the lye solution to ensure the correct chemical reaction and soap consistency.

✓ **Practice**: If you're new to soap making, practice safety protocols and follow established recipes closely to achieve desired results safely.

Preparing the lye solution is a crucial step in the liquid soap making process that requires careful attention to safety and precise measurements. By following these guidelines and safety precautions, you can effectively prepare a lye solution that forms the foundation for creating high-quality liquid soap products. Always prioritize safety, accuracy, and adherence to recommended procedures to achieve successful soap making outcomes.

4.2. Mixing Oils and Lye

Mixing oils and lye is a critical step in the liquid soap-making process. It's where the magic happens, turning your ingredients into a smooth, luscious soap. This part of the process requires precision, patience, and attention to safety. Here's a detailed, humanized guide to help you through it.

1. Preparing Your Ingredients

Before you start mixing, make sure all your ingredients are pre-measured and ready to go. This includes your oils, the lye solution, and any additives you plan to use.

1.1. Measure Your Oils

- ✓ **Oils and Fats**: Depending on your recipe, you'll need a mix of oils and fats. Common oils include olive oil, coconut oil, and castor oil. Weigh them out precisely using a digital scale.

✓ **Melt Solid Oils**: If you're using solid oils like coconut oil or shea butter, melt them gently in a double boiler until they're fully liquid.

1.2. Prepare the Lye Solution

✓ **Lye (Potassium Hydroxide)**: Ensure your lye solution is fully dissolved and has cooled to the appropriate temperature, as specified in your recipe.

2. Combining Oils and Lye

Now, let's combine the oils and the lye solution. This is where the real soap-making begins.

2.1. Safety First

✓ **Protective Gear**: Make sure you're wearing your rubber gloves, safety goggles, and an apron. Lye is caustic and can cause burns if it comes into contact with your skin.

✓ **Ventilation**: Work in a well-ventilated area to avoid inhaling any fumes.

2.2. Temperature Check

HOMEMADE LIQUID SOAP MAKING

- ✓ **Ideal Temperature**: Check the temperature of both the oils and the lye solution. They should be within the same temperature range, typically between 100°F and 130°F (38°C and 54°C), for optimal saponification.

- ✓ **Thermometer**: Use a digital thermometer to ensure accuracy.

2.3. Mixing Process

- ✓ **Pouring the Lye**: Slowly and carefully pour the lye solution into the oils. Pour in a steady stream while stirring gently.

- ✓ **Stick Blender**: Use a stick blender (immersion blender) to mix the oils and lye solution thoroughly. This helps achieve a uniform mixture and accelerates the saponification process.

- ✓ **Blend Until Trace**: Blend the mixture until it reaches "trace." Trace is when the soap mixture thickens to the point where you can drizzle a bit of it across the surface and it leaves a visible trail. This indicates that the oils and lye have emulsified properly.

3. Adding Additives

Once you've reached trace, it's time to add any fragrances, colorants, or other additives to your soap.

3.1. Fragrances

- ✓ **Essential Oils**: Add your chosen essential oils or fragrance oils. These not only give your soap a pleasant scent but also offer additional benefits like soothing or invigorating properties.

- ✓ **Measure Precisely**: Measure your fragrances accurately to avoid overpowering scents or irritation.

3.2. Colorants

- ✓ **Natural or Synthetic**: Choose between natural colorants (like clays or botanical powders) and synthetic ones. Mix them thoroughly to avoid streaks or uneven coloring.

- ✓ **Incorporate Fully**: Stir in the colorants until the soap has a uniform color.

3.3. Other Additives

- ✓ **Exfoliants**: Add exfoliating agents like ground oats, poppy seeds, or coffee grounds if you want your soap to have a scrubbing effect.

- ✓ **Moisturizers**: Enhance your soap with additional moisturizers like aloe vera gel or honey.

4. Transition to Cooking

With your oils and lye mixed and additives incorporated, you're ready to move on to the next phase—cooking the soap mixture.

4.1. Slow Cooker Method

- ✓ **Transfer to Slow Cooker**: Pour the soap mixture into a slow cooker. This method is known as the "hot process" and helps speed up the saponification.

- ✓ **Cook on Low Heat**: Set the slow cooker to a low heat setting and cover it.

- ✓ **Stir Occasionally**: Stir the soap occasionally to ensure even cooking.

4.2. Watch for Gel Phase

✓ **Gel Phase**: During cooking, the soap will enter a gel phase, where it becomes translucent and gel-like. This is a normal part of the process and indicates that saponification is occurring.

Mixing oils and lye is a transformative step in liquid soap making, requiring careful preparation and attention to detail. By following safety precautions, ensuring your ingredients are at the right temperature, and blending until you reach trace, you lay the foundation for a high-quality soap. Adding your personal touch with fragrances, colorants, and other additives makes the soap uniquely yours. With patience and precision, you'll master this process and create beautiful, homemade liquid soaps.

4.3. Achieving Trace

Achieving trace is a pivotal moment in the liquid soap-making process. It's when the oils and lye solution fully emulsify, creating a stable mixture that will eventually turn into soap. Understanding how to identify and achieve trace is crucial for successful soap making. Here's a detailed, humanized guide to help you navigate this essential step.

What is Trace?

HOMEMADE LIQUID SOAP MAKING

Definition: Trace is the point at which the oils and lye solution have mixed together sufficiently to form a thick, pudding-like consistency. It's called "trace" because you can see traces or trails of the mixture on the surface when you drizzle it back into the pot.

Importance: Reaching trace ensures that the saponification process (the chemical reaction that turns oils and lye into soap) is well underway and that the mixture is stable enough to add fragrances, colorants, and other additives without separating.

Steps to Achieve Trace

1. Preparation and Safety

Before you start mixing, ensure you have all your ingredients measured and your safety gear on.

- ✓ **Protective Gear**: Wear rubber gloves, safety goggles, and an apron to protect yourself from lye splashes.

- ✓ **Pre-measured Ingredients**: Have your oils, lye solution, and any additives ready and within reach.

2. Mixing Oils and Lye

2.1. Combine Oils and Lye Solution

HOMEMADE LIQUID SOAP MAKING

✓ **Slow and Steady**: Pour the lye solution into the oils slowly and steadily while stirring gently. This initial mixing can be done by hand to avoid splashes.

2.2. Use a Stick Blender

✓ **Immersion Blender**: A stick blender (also known as an immersion blender) is the best tool for achieving trace quickly and efficiently. It helps mix the oils and lye solution thoroughly, creating a smooth and uniform mixture.

✓ **Pulse and Stir**: Alternate between blending in short pulses and stirring by hand. This prevents the motor from overheating and ensures even mixing.

3. Identifying Trace

3.1. Thin Trace

✓ **Consistency**: The mixture will still be quite runny, similar to thin pancake batter. You'll notice a slight thickening, but it will still pour easily.

✓ **Use**: At this stage, you can incorporate lightweight additives like fragrances and colorants that blend easily without affecting the consistency too much.

3.2. Medium Trace

✓ **Consistency**: The mixture will thicken to a custard-like consistency. When you lift the blender or spoon, the mixture will leave noticeable trails on the surface.

✓ **Use**: This is the ideal stage to add heavier additives like exfoliants or botanicals, ensuring they are evenly distributed.

3.3. Thick Trace

✓ **Consistency**: The mixture is much thicker, resembling pudding. It will hold its shape on the surface and won't blend back in easily.

✓ **Use**: Achieving thick trace is necessary for certain designs or when you need the soap to set quickly in molds.

4. Tips for Achieving and Recognizing Trace

4.1. Patience and Observation

✓ **Watch Closely**: Keep a close eye on the consistency as you blend. It can change quickly, and it's easy to go from thin to thick trace without noticing.

✓ **Feel the Resistance**: You'll feel the mixture offer more resistance as it thickens. This is a good indicator that you're approaching trace.

4.2. Temperature Control

✓ **Monitor Temperatures**: Ensure your oils and lye solution are within the same temperature range, typically between 100°F and 130°F (38°C and 54°C). If the temperatures vary too much, it can affect how quickly you reach trace.

4.3. Practice and Experience

✓ **Trial and Error**: Achieving the perfect trace comes with practice. Don't be discouraged if it takes a few tries to get it right.

✓ **Learn from Each Batch**: Every batch of soap can teach you something new. Pay attention to how different oils and additives affect the tracing process.

Common Challenges and Solutions

1. Trace Taking Too Long

✓ **Problem**: If it seems to take forever to reach trace, it could be due to cooler temperatures or insufficient blending.

✓ **Solution**: Warm your oils and lye solution slightly and continue blending with the stick blender.

2. Trace Happening Too Quickly

✓ **Problem**: If your mixture thickens too quickly, it could be due to higher temperatures or certain additives that accelerate tracing.

✓ **Solution**: Work quickly and ensure your additives are ready to be incorporated as soon as you reach trace.

Achieving trace is a critical step in liquid soap making that requires careful attention and a bit of practice. By understanding the different stages of trace and how to recognize them, you can ensure a successful soap-making process. Use your stick blender wisely, monitor temperatures closely, and be patient. With time and experience, you'll master the art of reaching trace, paving the way for beautiful, high-quality liquid soaps.

4.4. Cooking the Soap

Cooking the soap is an integral part of the liquid soap-making process, especially if you are using the hot process method. This step ensures that the saponification process is complete and that your soap is ready for use sooner than with the cold process method. Here's a detailed guide on how to cook your soap, presented in a friendly, humanized tone.

Why Cook the Soap?

Speeding Up Saponification: Cooking the soap accelerates the saponification process, allowing the soap to be ready for use much sooner than the cold process method. **Ensuring Full Saponification**: By cooking the soap, you ensure that all the lye has reacted with the oils, resulting in a milder finished product.

1. Preparing to Cook the Soap

1.1. Gather Your Equipment

- ✓ **Slow Cooker**: A slow cooker is ideal for this step as it provides steady, even heat. Ensure it's clean and free of any residues.

- ✓ **Spatula or Spoon**: A heat-resistant spatula or spoon for stirring the soap.

✓ **Thermometer**: A digital thermometer to monitor the temperature of the soap mixture.

1.2. Safety First

✓ **Protective Gear**: Continue wearing your protective gear—rubber gloves, safety goggles, and an apron. Even though the mixture is more stable at this stage, it's still important to protect yourself from potential splashes.

2. Cooking the Soap

2.1. Transfer the Mixture

✓ **Pour Carefully**: Carefully pour the soap mixture into the slow cooker. Use your spatula to scrape out all the mixture from your mixing container to ensure none is wasted.

2.2. Set the Temperature

✓ **Low Heat**: Set the slow cooker to a low heat setting. This gentle heat is sufficient to cook the soap without causing it to overheat or scorch.

2.3. Stir Occasionally

✓ **Stir Gently**: Stir the soap mixture occasionally to ensure even cooking and to prevent it from sticking to the sides of the slow cooker. Use your spatula to scrape the sides and bottom to avoid any unmixed portions.

3. Monitoring the Cooking Process

3.1. Gel Phase

- ✓ **Visual Changes**: During cooking, the soap will go through various stages. It will first become more translucent and gel-like, which is known as the "gel phase." This is a sign that saponification is progressing.

- ✓ **Temperature Check**: Keep the temperature between 140°F and 180°F (60°C and 82°C). Use your thermometer to monitor the temperature and adjust the slow cooker settings if necessary.

3.2. "Vaseline" Stage

- ✓ **Consistency**: As cooking continues, the soap will thicken and take on a "Vaseline" or translucent appearance. This indicates that the saponification is nearing completion.

4. Testing for Completion

4.1. Clarity Test

✓ **Water Test**: Take a small spoonful of the soap mixture and dilute it in a cup of hot water. Stir it well. If the soap mixture dissolves and the water remains clear or slightly cloudy, the soap is done. If it's milky, it needs more cooking time.

4.2. pH Test

✓ **pH Strips**: Once you believe the soap is fully cooked, you can check its pH level using pH strips. A pH of 9-10 is typical for liquid soap, indicating it's ready.

5. Post-Cooking Steps

5.1. Dilution

✓ **Add Water**: If the soap is too thick, you may need to dilute it. Gradually add distilled water, stirring well, until you achieve the desired consistency. Be cautious not to add too much water at once; it's easier to thin the soap than to thicken it.

✓ **Consistency Check**: The soap should be pourable but not too watery. Aim for a honey-like consistency.

5.2. Adding Additives

✓ **Fragrances and Colorants**: If you haven't added fragrances or colorants earlier, now is the time. Add them slowly and stir well to ensure even distribution.

✓ **Preservatives**: If you're using natural additives that might spoil, consider adding a preservative suitable for liquid soap to extend its shelf life.

5.3. Cooling and Bottling

✓ **Cool the Soap**: Allow the soap to cool slightly in the slow cooker. Once it's safe to handle, pour it into clean, sterilized bottles or containers.

✓ **Label and Store**: Label your bottles with the date and ingredients. Store them in a cool, dry place.

Cooking the soap is a crucial step in the hot process method that ensures your liquid soap is fully saponified and ready for use. By carefully transferring the mixture to a slow cooker, monitoring its progress through the gel and "Vaseline" stages, and performing clarity and pH tests, you can create a high-quality liquid soap. With patience and attention to detail, you'll master this step, resulting in a beautifully crafted soap that's safe and effective for everyday use.

4.5. Dilution Process

The dilution process is the final critical step in making liquid soap. After cooking the soap to ensure full saponification, you'll need to dilute the thick soap paste to achieve the desired liquid consistency. This process requires patience and precision to get the right texture and clarity. Here's a detailed guide to help you through the dilution process in a humanized tone.

Understanding the Dilution Process

Why Dilute?

- ✓ **Achieve Liquid Consistency**: The soap paste created during the cooking phase is too thick to use as is. Diluting it turns the paste into a pourable liquid soap.

- ✓ **Control Viscosity**: Dilution allows you to adjust the soap's thickness to your preference, whether you want a thick, syrupy soap or a more fluid one.

Factors Affecting Dilution

- ✓ **Soap Recipe**: Different oil combinations create soap pastes that may require varying amounts of water for dilution.

- ✓ **Desired Consistency**: The final use of the soap (e.g., hand soap, body wash) will determine how much water you need to add.

1. Preparing for Dilution

1.1. Gather Equipment and Ingredients

- ✓ **Distilled Water**: Use distilled water to avoid impurities and ensure a clear soap. Tap water may contain minerals that can affect the clarity and performance of your soap.

- ✓ **Measuring Cups**: Accurate measurements are crucial for consistent results.

- ✓ **Large Pot or Slow Cooker**: For heating and mixing the soap paste and water.

- ✓ **Stick Blender**: To ensure thorough mixing of the soap paste and water.

1.2. Safety First

HOMEMADE LIQUID SOAP MAKING

✓ **Protective Gear**: Continue wearing your rubber gloves and safety goggles to protect against any potential splashes or spills.

2. Diluting the Soap Paste

2.1. Heating the Water

✓ **Warm Water**: Heat the distilled water to a temperature similar to the soap paste (around 120°F to 140°F or 49°C to 60°C). Warm water helps the soap paste dissolve more easily.

✓ **Avoid Boiling**: Do not boil the water, as too high a temperature can affect the soap's properties.

2.2. Adding Water to Soap Paste

✓ **Start Slowly**: Begin by adding a small amount of warm water to the soap paste. A good starting ratio is 1 part soap paste to 0.5-1 part water. You can always add more water later if needed.

✓ **Stir Gently**: Stir the mixture gently but thoroughly. A stick blender can be useful for breaking up the paste and ensuring an even consistency.

2.3. Letting the Soap Sit

✓ **Rest Period**: After the initial mixing, let the soap sit for several hours or overnight. This allows the soap paste to fully absorb the water.

✓ **Check Consistency**: After the resting period, check the soap's consistency. If it's too thick, gradually add more warm water, stirring gently each time, until you reach the desired consistency.

2.4. Final Adjustments

✓ **Consistency Check**: The soap should be smooth and pourable. For hand soap, a thinner consistency is often preferred, while for body wash, a slightly thicker texture might be desirable.

✓ **Clarity Test**: Your soap should be clear or only slightly cloudy. If it's too cloudy, you may need to adjust the dilution or check the quality of your water and ingredients.

3. Adding Finishing Touches

3.1. Fragrances and Essential Oils

✓ **Add Slowly**: If you haven't added fragrances or essential oils earlier, now is the time. Add them slowly, stirring thoroughly to ensure even distribution.

✓ **Test for Sensitivity**: Remember that some fragrances can cause the soap to thicken or thin out, so test with a small amount first.

3.2. Colorants and Additives

✓ **Incorporate Evenly**: If using colorants, mix them in thoroughly to avoid streaks or uneven coloring.

✓ **Additional Benefits**: Additives like aloe vera, vitamin E, or glycerin can enhance the soap's properties. Add them at this stage and mix well.

4. Bottling and Storing Your Soap

4.1. Bottling

✓ **Clean Containers**: Use clean, sterilized bottles or dispensers to store your soap. This helps prevent contamination and extends the shelf life of your soap.

✓ **Funnel for Precision**: Use a funnel to pour the soap into containers, minimizing spills and ensuring clean transfers.

4.2. Labeling

✓ **Accurate Labels**: Label each bottle with the type of soap, date of production, and ingredients used. This is especially useful if you're making multiple batches or variations.

4.3. Storage

✓ **Cool, Dark Place**: Store the bottled soap in a cool, dark place to preserve its quality. Proper storage helps maintain the soap's consistency and prevents the growth of bacteria or mold.

The dilution process is a vital step in making liquid soap, transforming the thick soap paste into a usable, pourable product. By carefully heating distilled water, gradually mixing it with the soap paste, and allowing time for absorption, you can achieve the perfect consistency. Adding final touches like fragrances and colorants, and ensuring proper bottling and storage, completes your liquid soap-making journey. With patience and attention to detail, you'll create a beautiful, high-quality liquid soap ready for everyday use.

4.6. Adding Fragrances and Colorants

Adding fragrances and colorants to your liquid soap is an exciting step that allows you to personalize your creation, making it unique and appealing. This step requires careful consideration of the types of additives you use and how they interact with your soap base. Here's a detailed guide to help you through the process in a humanized tone.

Why Add Fragrances and Colorants?

Enhance User Experience: Fragrances and colorants make your soap more enjoyable to use by adding pleasant scents and attractive colors. **Customization**: You can tailor the soap to your preferences or create different varieties for different purposes (e.g., soothing lavender for a calming hand soap or invigorating citrus for a refreshing body wash).

1. Choosing Fragrances

1.1. Types of Fragrances

✓ **Essential Oils**: Natural and derived from plants, essential oils offer a wide range of scents and additional benefits (e.g., lavender for relaxation, tea tree for antibacterial properties).

HOMEMADE LIQUID SOAP MAKING

✓ **Fragrance Oils**: Synthetic and often more stable in soap, fragrance oils come in an endless variety of scents, from floral to fruity to gourmand.

1.2. Considerations for Fragrance Selection

✓ **Allergies and Sensitivities**: Be mindful of potential allergens, especially if the soap is for sensitive skin or children.

✓ **Scent Strength**: Essential oils are typically more potent than fragrance oils. Start with a small amount and adjust as needed.

✓ **Combining Scents**: Experiment with blending different oils to create unique scent profiles. For example, mix lavender and eucalyptus for a spa-like aroma.

2. Adding Fragrances to Liquid Soap

2.1. When to Add Fragrance

✓ **After Dilution**: Add fragrances after the soap has been diluted and cooled slightly to prevent the volatile oils from evaporating due to heat.

2.2. How Much to Add

✓ **Recommended Amounts**: A general rule is to add 0.5-1% of the total soap weight in essential or fragrance oils. For example, if you have 1,000 grams of soap, add 5-10 grams of fragrance.

✓ **Start Small**: Begin with a lower amount, mix thoroughly, and then add more if needed. You can always add more, but you can't take it out once it's in.

2.3. Mixing Fragrances

✓ **Incorporate Evenly**: Stir the fragrance thoroughly into the soap to ensure even distribution. Use a stick blender or a spatula to mix well.

✓ **Check for Reaction**: Some fragrances can cause the soap to thicken or change color. Add a small amount first to see how it reacts before adding more.

3. Choosing Colorants

3.1. Types of Colorants

✓ **Natural Colorants**: Derived from plants and minerals, natural colorants include clays (e.g., rose clay), herbs (e.g., spirulina), and botanicals (e.g., turmeric).

✓ **Synthetic Colorants**: Include mica powders, liquid soap dyes, and FD&C colorants. They offer vibrant colors and are usually more stable.

3.2. Considerations for Colorant Selection

✓ **Skin Safety**: Ensure the colorants are skin-safe and suitable for soap making.

✓ **Stability**: Some natural colorants may fade over time or react with the soap's pH, altering the final color.

4. Adding Colorants to Liquid Soap

4.1. When to Add Colorants

✓ **Before Final Bottling**: Add colorants after dilution and before bottling to achieve even coloration throughout the batch.

4.2. How Much to Add

✓ **Recommended Amounts**: The amount varies depending on the type of colorant. Start with a small amount (e.g., 1/8 teaspoon of mica per pound of soap) and adjust as needed.

- ✓ **Mixing and Testing**: Mix a small batch first to test the color intensity. Remember that some colors may deepen as the soap cures.

4.3. Mixing Colorants

- ✓ **Pre-Dissolve if Necessary**: Some colorants, especially powders, should be pre-dissolved in a small amount of warm water or glycerin to prevent clumping.

- ✓ **Stir Thoroughly**: Mix the colorant evenly into the soap. Use a stick blender for thorough blending, especially if using powder colorants.

5. Troubleshooting Common Issues

5.1. Fragrance Fading

- ✓ **Solution**: Some essential oils, like citrus, tend to fade over time. Use fragrance oils or blend with fixative oils (e.g., cedarwood) to help the scent last longer.

5.2. Color Bleeding

- ✓ **Solution**: If colors start to bleed or migrate, it may be due to using too much colorant or unstable colorants. Reduce the amount and ensure the colorant is suitable for liquid soap.

5.3. Cloudy Soap

- ✓ **Solution**: Some colorants and fragrances can cause soap to become cloudy. Use distilled water, test additives in small batches, and avoid overuse of additives.

6. Final Steps

6.1. Bottling and Labeling

- ✓ **Clean Bottles**: Ensure your bottles or dispensers are clean and dry before filling.

- ✓ **Use a Funnel**: Use a funnel to pour the soap into bottles, minimizing spills.

- ✓ **Label Clearly**: Label each bottle with the scent and color, along with the production date and ingredients.

6.2. Storing Finished Soap

- ✓ **Cool, Dark Place**: Store the finished soap in a cool, dark place to preserve the fragrance and color.

✓ **Monitor Quality**: Check the soap periodically for any changes in scent or color.

Adding fragrances and colorants to your liquid soap allows you to create a product that's not only functional but also a delight to use. By carefully selecting and mixing your fragrances and colorants, you can customize your soap to suit your preferences and needs. Always test your additives in small batches first, ensure even distribution, and be mindful of any reactions. With these steps, you'll produce beautiful, aromatic, and visually appealing liquid soaps that are sure to be enjoyed by everyone.

4.7. Bottling and Storing

Bottling and storing your liquid soap is the final step in your soap-making journey. This stage is crucial for maintaining the quality and longevity of your product. Proper bottling ensures that your soap remains fresh and effective, while proper storage extends its shelf life and keeps it safe from contamination. Here's a detailed guide to help you through the bottling and storing process in a friendly, humanized tone.

Why Bottling and Storing Matter

Preserve Quality: Proper bottling and storage help maintain the soap's fragrance, color, and effectiveness over time. **Prevent Contamination**: Clean and sealed containers protect your soap from dust, bacteria, and other contaminants. **Convenience**: Bottling your soap in user-friendly containers makes it easy to use and dispense, adding to the overall user experience.

1. Choosing the Right Bottles

1.1. Bottle Types

- ✓ **Plastic Bottles**: Lightweight and shatterproof, plastic bottles are a popular choice. Opt for BPA-free plastic to ensure safety.

- ✓ **Glass Bottles**: Glass bottles offer a more upscale appearance and are better for essential oils, as they don't react with the contents. However, they are heavier and can break if dropped.

- ✓ **Pump Dispensers**: Ideal for hand soaps and lotions, pump dispensers provide ease of use.

- ✓ **Squeeze Bottles**: Great for body washes and shampoos, squeeze bottles offer controlled dispensing.

HOMEMADE LIQUID SOAP MAKING

1.2. Size Considerations

- ✓ **Small Bottles (2-4 oz)**: Good for travel sizes or samples.

- ✓ **Medium Bottles (8-16 oz)**: Ideal for daily use at home.

- ✓ **Large Bottles (32 oz and up)**: Suitable for refills or bulk storage.

2. Preparing for Bottling

2.1. Cleaning and Sterilizing

- ✓ **Wash Bottles**: Clean your bottles thoroughly with hot, soapy water. Rinse well to remove any soap residue.

- ✓ **Sterilize**: For added safety, sterilize the bottles by soaking them in a solution of 1 part bleach to 9 parts water, then rinse with boiling water. Let them air dry completely.

2.2. Tools and Accessories

- ✓ **Funnel**: A funnel makes it easier to pour the soap into bottles without spills.

✓ **Measuring Cups**: Use measuring cups to ensure consistent portions if you're dividing the soap into multiple containers.

✓ **Labels and Markers**: Have labels and markers ready for identifying and dating your soap.

3. Bottling the Soap

3.1. Pouring the Soap

✓ **Cool the Soap**: Ensure the soap is cool enough to handle safely, but not so cool that it becomes too thick to pour.

✓ **Use a Funnel**: Place a funnel in the mouth of the bottle and slowly pour the soap. Take care to pour steadily to avoid air bubbles.

✓ **Fill to Appropriate Level**: Leave a little space at the top of each bottle to allow for expansion and easy dispensing.

3.2. Sealing the Bottles

✓ **Secure Lids**: Immediately seal the bottles with their caps or pump dispensers to prevent contamination.

HOMEMADE LIQUID SOAP MAKING

- ✓ **Check for Leaks**: After sealing, check each bottle for leaks by gently tipping it upside down.

4. Labeling Your Soap

4.1. Essential Information

- ✓ **Name and Type**: Include the name of the soap and its type (e.g., lavender hand soap, citrus body wash).

- ✓ **Ingredients**: List all ingredients used, especially if you plan to sell the soap or give it as a gift.

- ✓ **Date**: Note the date of production so you can track its age and use it within a reasonable time frame.

4.2. Additional Details

- ✓ **Usage Instructions**: Provide any specific usage instructions, especially if the soap contains special additives or is intended for a particular use.

- ✓ **Allergen Warnings**: Highlight any potential allergens, such as essential oils or nut-based ingredients.

5. Storing Your Soap

5.1. Optimal Storage Conditions

- ✓ **Cool, Dark Place**: Store your bottled soap in a cool, dark place away from direct sunlight and heat sources. A cupboard or closet works well.

- ✓ **Avoid Moisture**: Keep the soap in a dry area to prevent mold and mildew growth.

5.2. Shelf Life

- ✓ **Typical Duration**: Properly stored liquid soap can last 6 months to a year. Some natural ingredients may reduce shelf life, so consider adding a natural preservative if needed.

- ✓ **Monitoring Quality**: Check your stored soap periodically for any changes in scent, color, or texture. If you notice any off smells, discoloration, or separation, it's best to discard the soap.

6. Tips for Long-Term Storage

6.1. Bulk Storage

- ✓ **Large Containers**: If you're making large batches, store the bulk soap in large, airtight containers. Decant into smaller bottles as needed.

- ✓ **Label Clearly**: Ensure each large container is labeled with the soap type and production date.

6.2. Preservatives

- ✓ **Natural Preservatives**: Consider using natural preservatives like vitamin E, grapefruit seed extract, or rosemary extract to extend shelf life without compromising the soap's natural qualities.

- ✓ **Synthetic Preservatives**: If you prefer longer shelf life, synthetic preservatives like Germaben II or Optiphen can be used, but follow recommended usage rates carefully.

Bottling and storing your liquid soap correctly is essential to maintaining its quality, safety, and usability. By choosing the right bottles, ensuring thorough cleaning and sterilization, carefully pouring and sealing the soap, and labeling it accurately, you can enjoy your handmade liquid soap for months to come. Proper storage conditions further enhance the soap's longevity, allowing you to savor the fruits of your labor in every wash.

CHAPTER FIVE

RECIPES FOR BEGINNERS

5.1. Simple Liquid Soap Recipe

Creating your own liquid soap at home can be both a rewarding and cost-effective endeavor, especially if you're new to soap making. This simple liquid soap recipe is designed for beginners, offering a straightforward process that produces a gentle and effective soap. Let's dive into the details and get you started on your soap-making journey.

Why Make Your Own Liquid Soap?

Customizable: You can tailor the ingredients to suit your preferences, skin type, and any allergies you may have. **Natural Ingredients**: Making your own soap allows you to avoid harsh chemicals and artificial additives found in many commercial soaps. **Cost-Effective**: Homemade soap can be more economical in the long run, especially if you make it in large batches. **Satisfaction**: There's a unique satisfaction in using a product you made yourself.

Ingredients for Simple Liquid Soap

To make this simple liquid soap, you'll need the following ingredients:

HOMEMADE LIQUID SOAP MAKING

1. **Distilled Water**: 32 ounces (950 ml)

2. **Oils and Fats**: This recipe uses a combination of olive oil and coconut oil for a balanced blend of moisturizing and cleansing properties.

   - ✓ **Olive Oil**: 12 ounces (340 grams)

   - ✓ **Coconut Oil**: 8 ounces (225 grams)

3. **Potassium Hydroxide (KOH)**: 4.5 ounces (125 grams). This is the lye needed for liquid soap. Make sure to use potassium hydroxide, not sodium hydroxide (NaOH).

4. **Glycerin**: 2 ounces (60 ml). Glycerin adds moisture and improves the transparency of the soap.

5. **Essential Oils** (optional): About 1-2 teaspoons (5-10 ml), depending on your preference. Some popular choices include lavender, peppermint, or tea tree oil.

Equipment Needed

1. **Safety Gear**: Gloves, safety goggles, and a long-sleeved shirt to protect against lye splashes.

2. **Stainless Steel or Heat-Resistant Plastic Mixing Bowl**: For mixing the lye solution.

HOMEMADE LIQUID SOAP MAKING

3. **Stick Blender**: For blending the soap mixture.

4. **Stainless Steel or Heavy-Duty Plastic Pot**: For cooking the soap.

5. **Heat-Resistant Spoon or Spatula**: For stirring.

6. **Digital Scale**: For accurately measuring ingredients.

7. **Thermometer**: To monitor the temperature of the lye solution and oils.

8. **Measuring Cups and Spoons**: For measuring water, glycerin, and essential oils.

9. **Containers for Soap Storage**: Clean bottles or jars to store the finished soap.

Step-by-Step Instructions

Step 1: Prepare Your Workspace

1. **Set Up**: Choose a well-ventilated area to work in. Cover your workspace with newspaper or a protective mat to catch any spills.

2. **Gather Equipment and Ingredients**: Ensure you have everything you need within reach before you begin.

Step 2: Make the Lye Solution

1. **Safety First**: Put on your gloves, safety goggles, and long-sleeved shirt.

2. **Weigh Water and Potassium Hydroxide**: Using your digital scale, measure 32 ounces (950 ml) of distilled water and 4.5 ounces (125 grams) of potassium hydroxide.

3. **Mix Carefully**: Slowly add the potassium hydroxide to the distilled water, stirring gently. Never add water to lye, as it can cause a dangerous reaction. The mixture will heat up quickly. Stir until the potassium hydroxide is completely dissolved, then set aside to cool.

Step 3: Weigh and Melt the Oils

1. **Measure Oils**: Weigh out 12 ounces (340 grams) of olive oil and 8 ounces (225 grams) of coconut oil.

2. **Melt Coconut Oil**: In a stainless steel or heavy-duty plastic pot, gently heat the coconut oil until it melts. Add the olive oil and mix thoroughly.

HOMEMADE LIQUID SOAP MAKING

Step 4: Combine Oils and Lye Solution

1. **Check Temperatures**: Ensure that both the lye solution and the oils are around 120°F (49°C) to 140°F (60°C).

2. **Mix Together**: Slowly pour the lye solution into the pot with the oils, stirring continuously.

Step 5: Blend to Trace

1. **Use Stick Blender**: Using a stick blender, blend the mixture until it reaches "trace." Trace is when the mixture thickens and leaves a trail on the surface when dripped from a spoon.

2. **Add Glycerin**: Once trace is achieved, add 2 ounces (60 ml) of glycerin and blend thoroughly.

Step 6: Cook the Soap

1. **Cook on Low Heat**: Place the pot on low heat and cook the soap mixture. Stir occasionally.

2. **Gel Phase**: The soap will go through a gel phase, becoming translucent. This can take 1-2 hours.

3. **Test Clarity**: To check if the soap is done, dissolve a small amount in hot water. If the solution is clear, the soap is ready. If it's cloudy, continue cooking.

HOMEMADE LIQUID SOAP MAKING

Step 7: Dilute the Soap Paste

1. **Dilute with Water**: Once the soap paste is fully cooked, it's time to dilute. Add the remaining distilled water gradually, stirring continuously until the desired consistency is reached. For this recipe, you'll need about 32 ounces (950 ml) of water.

2. **Optional: Add Essential Oils**: If you're adding essential oils, now is the time. Add about 1-2 teaspoons (5-10 ml) and stir well.

Step 8: Cool and Bottle

1. **Cool the Soap**: Allow the soap to cool slightly before transferring it to storage containers.

2. **Bottle the Soap**: Use a funnel to pour the soap into clean bottles or jars. Seal the containers and label them with the date and type of soap.

Step 9: Store and Enjoy

1. **Storage**: Store the soap in a cool, dark place. Properly stored, the soap can last for 6 months to a year.

2. **Use and Share**: Enjoy your homemade liquid soap and share it with friends and family!

This simple liquid soap recipe is perfect for beginners, offering a straightforward process and a satisfying end product. By following these steps, you can create a gentle, effective soap tailored to your preferences. With practice, you'll gain confidence and may even start experimenting with different oils, scents, and colors. Happy soap making!

5.2. Moisturizing Liquid Soap

For those who have dry or sensitive skin, a moisturizing liquid soap can make all the difference in maintaining soft, hydrated hands and body. This recipe incorporates nourishing ingredients that cleanse without stripping your skin of its natural oils. Here's an extensive guide to creating your own moisturizing liquid soap, complete with tips and techniques to ensure a smooth and successful soap-making experience.

Benefits of Moisturizing Liquid Soap

Hydration: Contains ingredients that add moisture to the skin, preventing dryness and irritation. **Nourishment**: Enriched with oils and butters that provide essential nutrients and antioxidants. **Gentle Cleansing**: Effectively cleanses without harsh chemicals, making it suitable for sensitive skin. **Customization**: Allows you to tailor the recipe to your specific skin needs and preferences.

Ingredients for Moisturizing Liquid Soap

To create a moisturizing liquid soap, you'll need the following ingredients:

1. **Distilled Water**: 32 ounces (950 ml)

2. **Oils and Butters**: This recipe uses a combination of olive oil, coconut oil, and shea butter for their moisturizing and nourishing properties.

   ✓ **Olive Oil**: 10 ounces (285 grams)

   ✓ **Coconut Oil**: 8 ounces (225 grams)

   ✓ **Shea Butter**: 4 ounces (115 grams)

3. **Potassium Hydroxide (KOH)**: 4.5 ounces (125 grams)

4. **Glycerin**: 2 ounces (60 ml). Glycerin is a humectant that draws moisture to the skin.

5. **Essential Oils** (optional): About 1-2 teaspoons (5-10 ml) of skin-soothing essential oils like lavender, chamomile, or geranium.

HOMEMADE LIQUID SOAP MAKING

Equipment Needed

1. **Safety Gear**: Gloves, safety goggles, and a long-sleeved shirt to protect against lye splashes.

2. **Stainless Steel or Heat-Resistant Plastic Mixing Bowl**: For mixing the lye solution.

3. **Stick Blender**: For blending the soap mixture.

4. **Stainless Steel or Heavy-Duty Plastic Pot**: For cooking the soap.

5. **Heat-Resistant Spoon or Spatula**: For stirring.

6. **Digital Scale**: For accurately measuring ingredients.

7. **Thermometer**: To monitor the temperature of the lye solution and oils.

8. **Measuring Cups and Spoons**: For measuring water, glycerin, and essential oils.

9. **Containers for Soap Storage**: Clean bottles or jars to store the finished soap.

HOMEMADE LIQUID SOAP MAKING

Step-by-Step Instructions

Step 1: Prepare Your Workspace

1. **Set Up**: Choose a well-ventilated area to work in. Cover your workspace with newspaper or a protective mat to catch any spills.

2. **Gather Equipment and Ingredients**: Ensure you have everything you need within reach before you begin.

Step 2: Make the Lye Solution

1. **Safety First**: Put on your gloves, safety goggles, and long-sleeved shirt.

2. **Weigh Water and Potassium Hydroxide**: Using your digital scale, measure 32 ounces (950 ml) of distilled water and 4.5 ounces (125 grams) of potassium hydroxide.

3. **Mix Carefully**: Slowly add the potassium hydroxide to the distilled water, stirring gently. Never add water to lye, as it can cause a dangerous reaction. The mixture will heat up quickly. Stir until the potassium hydroxide is completely dissolved, then set aside to cool.

HOMEMADE LIQUID SOAP MAKING

Step 3: Weigh and Melt the Oils and Butters

1. **Measure Oils and Butter**: Weigh out 10 ounces (285 grams) of olive oil, 8 ounces (225 grams) of coconut oil, and 4 ounces (115 grams) of shea butter.

2. **Melt Coconut Oil and Shea Butter**: In a stainless steel or heavy-duty plastic pot, gently heat the coconut oil and shea butter until they melt. Add the olive oil and mix thoroughly.

Step 4: Combine Oils and Lye Solution

1. **Check Temperatures**: Ensure that both the lye solution and the oils are around 120°F (49°C) to 140°F (60°C).

2. **Mix Together**: Slowly pour the lye solution into the pot with the oils, stirring continuously.

Step 5: Blend to Trace

1. **Use Stick Blender**: Using a stick blender, blend the mixture until it reaches "trace." Trace is when the mixture thickens and leaves a trail on the surface when dripped from a spoon.

2. **Add Glycerin**: Once trace is achieved, add 2 ounces (60 ml) of glycerin and blend thoroughly.

Step 6: Cook the Soap

1. **Cook on Low Heat**: Place the pot on low heat and cook the soap mixture. Stir occasionally.

2. **Gel Phase**: The soap will go through a gel phase, becoming translucent. This can take 1-2 hours.

3. **Test Clarity**: To check if the soap is done, dissolve a small amount in hot water. If the solution is clear, the soap is ready. If it's cloudy, continue cooking.

Step 7: Dilute the Soap Paste

1. **Dilute with Water**: Once the soap paste is fully cooked, it's time to dilute. Add the remaining distilled water gradually, stirring continuously until the desired consistency is reached. For this recipe, you'll need about 32 ounces (950 ml) of water.

2. **Optional: Add Essential Oils**: If you're adding essential oils, now is the time. Add about 1-2 teaspoons (5-10 ml) and stir well.

Step 8: Cool and Bottle

HOMEMADE LIQUID SOAP MAKING

1. **Cool the Soap**: Allow the soap to cool slightly before transferring it to storage containers.

2. **Bottle the Soap**: Use a funnel to pour the soap into clean bottles or jars. Seal the containers and label them with the date and type of soap.

Step 9: Store and Enjoy

1. **Storage**: Store the soap in a cool, dark place. Properly stored, the soap can last for 6 months to a year.

2. **Use and Share**: Enjoy your homemade moisturizing liquid soap and share it with friends and family!

Tips for Customizing Your Moisturizing Liquid Soap

Choosing Essential Oils

- ✓ **Lavender**: Known for its calming and soothing properties, perfect for sensitive skin.

- ✓ **Chamomile**: Gentle and anti-inflammatory, great for irritated skin.

- ✓ **Geranium**: Balances skin oils and promotes a healthy complexion.

HOMEMADE LIQUID SOAP MAKING

Adding Botanical Extracts

- ✓ **Aloe Vera**: Adds extra moisture and soothes the skin.

- ✓ **Calendula**: Provides healing properties and is gentle on sensitive skin.

Using Hydrating Additives

- ✓ **Honey**: A natural humectant that attracts moisture to the skin.

- ✓ **Oat Milk**: Soothes and nourishes dry, itchy skin.

Creating a moisturizing liquid soap at home is a rewarding project that results in a gentle, nourishing product perfect for daily use. By carefully selecting and combining oils, butters, and other moisturizing ingredients, you can craft a soap that not only cleanses but also pampers your skin. Whether you choose to add essential oils, botanical extracts, or hydrating additives, this customizable recipe offers endless possibilities to suit your specific needs. Enjoy the process and the satisfaction of using a product made with care and tailored just for you.

5.3. Antibacterial Liquid Soap

Creating your own antibacterial liquid soap at home provides a customized solution for maintaining cleanliness and hygiene. This recipe incorporates effective antibacterial agents while ensuring gentle cleansing and skin nourishment. Here's an extensive guide to crafting your own antibacterial liquid soap, complete with ingredients, equipment, and step-by-step instructions to help you achieve a successful soap-making experience.

Antibacterial Liquid Soap

Antibacterial liquid soap serves as a valuable addition to your daily hygiene routine, providing effective germ protection without harsh chemicals. This recipe focuses on combining potent antibacterial ingredients with moisturizing elements to ensure clean and nourished skin. Let's explore how to create your own antibacterial liquid soap at home.

Benefits of Antibacterial Liquid Soap

- ✓ **Germ Protection**: Contains antibacterial agents that help eliminate harmful germs and bacteria.

HOMEMADE LIQUID SOAP MAKING

- ✓ **Gentle Formulation**: Designed to cleanse effectively without drying out the skin.

- ✓ **Customizable**: Allows you to tailor the ingredients to address specific skin concerns and preferences.

- ✓ **Cost-Effective**: Making your own soap can be more economical than purchasing commercial antibacterial products.

Ingredients for Antibacterial Liquid Soap

To make antibacterial liquid soap, gather the following ingredients:

1. **Distilled Water**: 32 ounces (950 ml)

2. **Oils and Butters**: This recipe uses a combination of coconut oil and olive oil for their cleansing and moisturizing properties.

   - ✓ **Coconut Oil**: 10 ounces (285 grams)

   - ✓ **Olive Oil**: 8 ounces (225 grams)

3. **Potassium Hydroxide (KOH)**: 4.5 ounces (125 grams)

4. **Glycerin**: 2 ounces (60 ml). Glycerin helps retain moisture and improves the soap's texture.

5. **Tea Tree Essential Oil**: 1-2 teaspoons (5-10 ml). Known for its antibacterial and antifungal properties.

6. **Lavender Essential Oil** (optional): 1 teaspoon (5 ml). Adds a pleasant scent and enhances the antibacterial properties.

Equipment Needed

Ensure you have the following equipment ready before starting:

1. **Safety Gear**: Gloves, safety goggles, and a long-sleeved shirt to protect against lye splashes.

2. **Stainless Steel or Heat-Resistant Plastic Mixing Bowl**: For mixing the lye solution.

3. **Stick Blender**: For blending the soap mixture.

4. **Stainless Steel or Heavy-Duty Plastic Pot**: For cooking the soap.

5. **Heat-Resistant Spoon or Spatula**: For stirring.

6. **Digital Scale**: For accurately measuring ingredients.

7. **Thermometer**: To monitor the temperature of the lye solution and oils.

8. **Measuring Cups and Spoons**: For measuring water, glycerin, and essential oils.

9. **Containers for Soap Storage**: Clean bottles or jars to store the finished soap.

Step-by-Step Instructions

Step 1: Prepare Your Workspace

- ✓ Choose a well-ventilated area and cover your workspace with newspaper or a protective mat.

Step 2: Make the Lye Solution

1. **Safety First**: Put on gloves, safety goggles, and a long-sleeved shirt.

2. **Weigh Water and Potassium Hydroxide**: Measure 32 ounces (950 ml) of distilled water and 4.5 ounces (125 grams) of potassium hydroxide.

3. **Mix Carefully**: Slowly add potassium hydroxide to distilled water, stirring gently. Avoid splashing. Stir until fully dissolved and set aside to cool.

Step 3: Weigh and Melt the Oils

1. **Measure Oils**: Weigh 10 ounces (285 grams) of coconut oil and 8 ounces (225 grams) of olive oil.

2. **Melt Coconut Oil**: In a stainless steel or heavy-duty plastic pot, gently heat coconut oil until it melts. Add olive oil and mix thoroughly.

Step 4: Combine Oils and Lye Solution

1. **Check Temperatures**: Ensure oils and lye solution are between 120°F (49°C) to 140°F (60°C).

2. **Mix Together**: Slowly pour lye solution into pot with oils, stirring continuously.

Step 5: Blend to Trace

1. **Use Stick Blender**: Blend mixture until it reaches "trace," leaving a trail on surface when dripped from spoon.

2. **Add Glycerin**: Once trace is achieved, add 2 ounces (60 ml) of glycerin and blend thoroughly.

Step 6: Cook the Soap

1. **Cook on Low Heat**: Place pot on low heat and cook soap mixture, stirring occasionally.

2. **Gel Phase**: Soap will go through gel phase, becoming translucent. This can take 1-2 hours.

3. **Test Clarity**: To check if soap is done, dissolve small amount in hot water. If clear, soap is ready. If cloudy, continue cooking.

Step 7: Dilute the Soap Paste

1. **Dilute with Water**: Once fully cooked, gradually add remaining distilled water, stirring continuously until desired consistency. For recipe, use about 32 ounces (950 ml) of water.

2. **Optional: Add Essential Oils**: Add 1-2 teaspoons (5-10 ml) of tea tree essential oil and 1 teaspoon (5 ml) of lavender essential oil. Stir well.

Step 8: Cool and Bottle

1. **Cool Soap**: Allow soap to cool slightly before transferring to storage containers.

2. **Bottle Soap**: Use funnel to pour soap into clean bottles or jars. Seal containers and label with date and type of soap.

Step 9: Store and Use

1. **Storage**: Store soap in cool, dark place. Properly stored, soap can last 6 months to 1 year.

HOMEMADE LIQUID SOAP MAKING

2. **Usage**: Enjoy your homemade antibacterial liquid soap for daily cleansing and germ protection.

Tips for Customizing Your Antibacterial Liquid Soap

- ✓ **Adjust Essential Oils**: Experiment with different antibacterial essential oils, such as eucalyptus, peppermint, or lemongrass, for varying scents and properties.

- ✓ **Enhance Moisture**: Include moisturizing additives like aloe vera gel or vitamin E oil to soothe and hydrate skin.

- ✓ **Natural Colorants**: Add natural colorants like turmeric or spirulina powder for aesthetic appeal without synthetic dyes.

Creating your own antibacterial liquid soap at home allows you to customize your hygiene routine with a gentle yet effective product. By combining antibacterial agents with nourishing oils and moisturizers, you can cleanse and protect your skin while avoiding harsh chemicals found in many commercial soaps. Whether for personal use or as a thoughtful gift, homemade antibacterial liquid soap offers peace of mind and promotes overall skin health. Enjoy the process of crafting your soap and the satisfaction of using a product tailored to your needs.

CHAPTER SIX

ADVANCED TECHNIQUES AND TIPS FOR SENIORS

6.1. Customizing Soap Formulas

Creating customized soap formulas for seniors involves tailoring ingredients and techniques to address age-related skin changes, preferences, and sensitivities. Whether it's adjusting moisturizing properties, incorporating soothing additives, or enhancing fragrance options, these advanced techniques ensure that seniors can enjoy safe, effective, and enjoyable soap products.

Understanding Seniors' Skin Needs

As we age, our skin undergoes several changes that can affect its texture, moisture levels, and sensitivity. Customizing soap formulas for seniors takes these factors into account to provide gentle cleansing and nourishment. Common considerations include:

- ✓ **Dryness**: Aging skin tends to become drier due to reduced oil production. Soap formulas should prioritize moisturizing ingredients to prevent dehydration and maintain skin elasticity.

✓ **Sensitive Skin**: Seniors may develop increased skin sensitivity, making them prone to irritation or allergic reactions. Choosing gentle, hypoallergenic ingredients helps minimize potential skin discomfort.

✓ **Fragrance Preferences**: Preferences for fragrance may change with age. Some seniors may prefer mild scents or fragrance-free options to avoid overwhelming smells that can trigger sensitivities.

Advanced Techniques for Customizing Soap Formulas

1. **Moisturizing Formulas**:

   ✓ **Ingredients**: Incorporate rich oils and butters such as shea butter, cocoa butter, or avocado oil to boost hydration and nourishment.

   ✓ **Additives**: Include moisturizing additives like glycerin, aloe vera gel, or oatmeal to soothe dry, irritated skin.

   ✓ **Essential Oils**: Choose gentle essential oils like lavender, chamomile, or geranium for their calming and skin-soothing properties.

2. **Sensitive Skin Formulas**:

    ✓ **Ingredients**: Opt for mild oils such as olive oil, almond oil, or sunflower oil that are less likely to cause irritation.

    ✓ **Additives**: Consider incorporating colloidal oatmeal, calendula extract, or chamomile tea for their anti-inflammatory and soothing benefits.

    ✓ **Fragrance-Free Options**: Offer unscented varieties or use minimal amounts of fragrance to cater to sensitive noses.

3. **Anti-Aging Formulas**:

    ✓ **Ingredients**: Include ingredients rich in antioxidants and vitamins, such as vitamin E, green tea extract, or rosehip oil, to combat signs of aging and promote skin renewal.

    ✓ **Exfoliation**: Gentle exfoliants like finely ground oatmeal or poppy seeds can help remove dead skin cells and promote a smoother complexion.

✓ **Firming Agents**: Consider adding ingredients like coffee grounds or clay to enhance skin firmness and elasticity.

4. **Aromatherapy Formulas**:

✓ **Ingredients**: Create blends with essential oils known for their therapeutic benefits, such as peppermint for energizing, lavender for relaxation, or citrus oils for mood enhancement.

✓ **Custom Blends**: Tailor aromatherapy blends based on seniors' preferences and desired therapeutic effects, ensuring a personalized sensory experience.

Tips for Crafting Customized Soap Formulas

✓ **Patch Testing**: Always conduct a patch test before using a new soap formula to check for potential allergic reactions or sensitivities.

✓ **Consultation**: Consult with seniors or their caregivers to understand specific skin concerns, fragrance preferences, and any allergies or sensitivities.

✓ **Labeling**: Clearly label soap products with ingredients and usage instructions to ensure seniors can make informed choices and use the product safely.

✓ **Storage**: Store homemade soap in a cool, dry place away from direct sunlight to preserve its quality and efficacy over time.

Customizing soap formulas for seniors involves combining advanced techniques with thoughtful ingredient selection to create products that prioritize skin health, comfort, and enjoyment. By understanding seniors' unique skin needs and preferences, soap makers can craft personalized formulas that promote hydration, soothe sensitive skin, and provide a pleasant sensory experience. Whether for personal use or as a thoughtful gift, customized soap formulas contribute to seniors' overall well-being and enhance their daily skincare routines.

6.2. Troubleshooting Common Issues

Troubleshooting common issues in soap making for seniors involves identifying and addressing challenges that may arise during the soap-making process. By understanding potential problems and implementing effective solutions, you can ensure the creation of high-quality, safe, and enjoyable soap products tailored to seniors' needs. Here's an extensive guide to troubleshooting common issues in soap making:

Common Issues in Soap Making

1. **Soap Separation or Ricing**:

   - ✓ **Cause**: Inadequate mixing of oils and lye solution, incorrect temperatures, or using incompatible ingredients.

   - ✓ **Solution**: Ensure thorough mixing of oils and lye solution until they reach trace. Monitor temperatures carefully and avoid drastic temperature differences between ingredients. Use compatible oils and additives.

2. **Incomplete Saponification**:

- ✓ **Cause**: Insufficient mixing time, inaccurate measurement of ingredients, or improper ratios of oils to lye.

- ✓ **Solution**: Extend mixing time until trace is achieved, ensuring all ingredients are thoroughly blended. Double-check measurements and follow recommended ratios for oils and lye.

3. **Soft or Sticky Soap**:

- ✓ **Cause**: Overdosing on soft oils or butters, inadequate curing time, or using too much water in the recipe.

- ✓ **Solution**: Adjust the recipe by reducing soft oils or butters and increasing harder oils like coconut or palm oil. Allow soap to cure longer, typically 4-6 weeks, to harden and improve texture. Ensure water amount follows recommended ratios for a balanced soap formula.

4. **Fragrance or Essential Oil Discoloration**:

- ✓ **Cause**: Essential oils reacting with lye or additives containing natural pigments.

✓ **Solution**: Choose essential oils that are stable and less likely to discolor, such as lavender or citrus oils. Test additives for compatibility with soap-making ingredients to avoid unexpected color changes.

5. **Soap Cracking or Breaking**:

   ✓ **Cause**: Rapid cooling of soap, uneven distribution of additives, or unmolding too soon.

   ✓ **Solution**: Allow soap to cool gradually at room temperature or in a controlled environment. Ensure even distribution of additives throughout the soap mixture. Follow recommended unmolding times to prevent premature cracking or breaking.

6. **Skin Irritation or Sensitivity**:

   ✓ **Cause**: Using harsh or allergenic ingredients, inadequate rinsing of lye solution, or insufficient curing time.

   ✓ **Solution**: Choose gentle, hypoallergenic ingredients suitable for sensitive skin. Rinse lye solution thoroughly from soap mixture to reduce residual irritation. Allow soap to cure fully to neutralize lye and stabilize ingredients for safe use.

Advanced Troubleshooting Tips

✓ **Adjusting Recipes**: Modify soap recipes by altering ingredient ratios or types to achieve desired characteristics, such as hardness, lather, or moisturization.

✓ **Testing and Documentation**: Conduct small-scale tests or batches to troubleshoot specific issues before scaling production. Keep detailed records of ingredients, methods, and outcomes to refine soap-making techniques over time.

✓ **Consulting Resources**: Refer to reputable soap-making resources, forums, or workshops for guidance on advanced techniques and troubleshooting tips from experienced soap makers.

Troubleshooting common issues in soap making for seniors involves proactive problem-solving and attention to detail throughout the soap-making process. By addressing challenges such as soap separation, incomplete saponification, or fragrance discoloration with effective solutions, you can ensure the creation of high-quality, safe, and enjoyable soap products tailored to meet the unique needs and preferences of seniors. Through continuous learning and adaptation of soap-making techniques, you can refine your skills and produce personalized soap formulas that promote skin health, comfort, and satisfaction for seniors.

6.3. Creative Additives and Variations

Exploring creative additives and variations in soap making allows for the customization of soap formulas to cater specifically to seniors' preferences and skin care needs. By incorporating innovative ingredients and techniques, soap makers can enhance the functionality, aesthetics, and therapeutic benefits of their products. Here's an extensive guide to creative additives and variations in soap making for seniors:

Benefits of Creative Additives

✓ **Enhanced Moisturization**: Ingredients like shea butter, cocoa butter, or avocado oil provide deep hydration, ideal for seniors with dry or sensitive skin.

✓ **Therapeutic Effects**: Essential oils such as lavender, chamomile, or tea tree offer calming, anti-inflammatory, and antibacterial properties, promoting skin health and relaxation.

✓ **Visual Appeal**: Natural colorants like turmeric, spirulina, or clay add visual interest without synthetic dyes, appealing to seniors with aesthetic preferences.

Creative Additives and Variations

1. **Moisturizing Additives**:

   ✓ **Shea Butter**: Rich in vitamins and fatty acids, shea butter deeply moisturizes and softens the skin.

   ✓ **Cocoa Butter**: Provides a protective barrier and improves skin elasticity.

   ✓ **Avocado Oil**: Contains vitamins A, D, and E, offering nourishment and enhancing skin texture.

   ✓ **Glycerin**: Acts as a humectant, attracting moisture to the skin and improving soap's lather and texture.

2. **Therapeutic Essential Oils**:

   ✓ **Lavender**: Known for its calming and soothing properties, ideal for promoting relaxation and reducing stress.

   ✓ **Chamomile**: Anti-inflammatory and gentle, suitable for sensitive skin and promoting overall skin health.

   ✓ **Tea Tree**: Antibacterial and antifungal, beneficial for cleansing and maintaining skin hygiene.

3. **Exfoliating Additives**:

   ✓ **Oatmeal**: Soothes and gently exfoliates, ideal for sensitive or aging skin.

   ✓ **Poppy Seeds**: Provides gentle exfoliation to remove dead skin cells and promote smoother skin texture.

   ✓ **Coffee Grounds**: Offers natural exfoliation and helps improve circulation.

4. **Visual and Aesthetic Additives**:

✓ **Natural Colorants**: Add botanical powders like turmeric (yellow), spirulina (green), or pink clay for subtle color variations.

✓ **Botanicals**: Incorporate dried herbs, flower petals, or seaweed for texture and visual appeal.

Innovative Techniques and Variations

✓ **Layered Soaps**: Create visually appealing layers using different colored soap batters or embedments for a multi-dimensional effect.

✓ **Swirl Designs**: Use swirling techniques with contrasting colors or additives like activated charcoal for artistic patterns.

✓ **Milk-Based Soaps**: Substitute water with milk (such as goat milk or almond milk) for added creaminess and skin benefits.

✓ **Custom Blends**: Experiment with unique combinations of essential oils, additives, and colorants to create signature soap blends tailored to seniors' preferences.

Tips for Using Creative Additives

- ✓ **Measure Accurately**: Follow recommended guidelines for adding additives to maintain soap stability and effectiveness.

- ✓ **Test Small Batches**: Conduct small-scale tests to assess the performance and skin compatibility of new additives or variations before full-scale production.

- ✓ **Documentation**: Keep detailed records of ingredient proportions, techniques, and outcomes for future reference and refinement of soap-making processes.

Exploring creative additives and variations in soap making for seniors enables soap makers to craft personalized products that address specific skin care needs, preferences, and aesthetic preferences. By incorporating moisturizing agents, therapeutic essential oils, exfoliating additives, and visual enhancements, you can enhance the functionality and appeal of homemade soaps. Through experimentation, innovation, and attention to detail, you can create high-quality, customized soap formulas that promote skin health, comfort, and satisfaction for seniors. Enjoy the process of crafting unique soap creations that cater to individual preferences and contribute to a positive skincare experience.

6.4. Scaling Up Production

Scaling up production in soap making involves increasing batch sizes and optimizing processes to meet larger demand while maintaining product quality and consistency. This section explores essential considerations, strategies, and tips for successfully scaling up soap production for seniors:

Benefits of Scaling Up Production

- ✓ **Efficiency**: Producing larger batches reduces per-unit costs and labor intensity, making soap making more cost-effective.

- ✓ **Consistency**: Streamlining processes ensures consistent product quality and meets growing demand.

- ✓ **Market Expansion**: Scaling up allows for increased product availability and potential for reaching a broader customer base.

Considerations for Scaling Up

1. **Equipment and Workspace**

- ✓ **Invest in Larger Equipment**: Upgrade to larger mixing containers, molds, and storage solutions suitable for increased batch sizes.

- ✓ **Workspace Optimization**: Arrange workspace for efficient workflow and accommodate larger equipment and storage needs.

2. **Ingredient Sourcing and Storage**

- ✓ **Bulk Purchasing**: Source ingredients in bulk to reduce costs and ensure consistent quality.

- ✓ **Proper Storage**: Store bulk ingredients in a cool, dry place to maintain freshness and prevent contamination.

3. **Process Standardization**

- ✓ **Document Procedures**: Create standardized operating procedures (SOPs) for each soap-making step to ensure consistency and quality control.

✓ **Training**: Train staff or volunteers on SOPs to maintain uniformity in production processes.

4. **Quality Control**

✓ **Batch Testing**: Implement batch testing protocols to monitor product quality, including pH levels, fragrance intensity, and visual appearance.

✓ **Feedback Mechanism**: Establish a feedback loop with customers or testers to gather insights and address any quality issues promptly.

Strategies for Efficient Production

1. **Batch Planning and Scheduling**

✓ **Production Schedule**: Develop a production schedule based on demand forecasts and market trends.

✓ **Batch Size Optimization**: Determine optimal batch sizes that balance efficiency with quality assurance.

2. **Workflow Optimization**

- ✓ **Lean Manufacturing Principles**: Apply lean principles to streamline workflows, minimize waste, and maximize efficiency.

- ✓ **Batch Processing**: Organize tasks in sequential order to optimize time and resource utilization.

3. **Safety and Compliance**

- ✓ **Regulatory Compliance**: Ensure compliance with local health and safety regulations, including proper labeling and ingredient disclosure.

- ✓ **Safety Protocols**: Maintain rigorous safety protocols for handling chemicals and equipment to protect workers and ensure product integrity.

Tips for Successful Scaling Up

- ✓ **Gradual Expansion**: Start with incremental increases in batch sizes to assess scalability and identify potential challenges.

✓ **Supplier Relationships**: Build strong relationships with reliable suppliers to secure consistent ingredient quality and availability.

✓ **Customer Communication**: Inform customers about production scale-up to manage expectations and maintain transparency.

Scaling up production in soap making for seniors involves strategic planning, process optimization, and adherence to quality standards. By investing in equipment, standardizing processes, and optimizing workflows, soap makers can efficiently meet growing demand while maintaining product quality and consistency. Through careful planning and implementation of scalable strategies, you can expand your soap-making operations to serve a broader audience of seniors, contributing to their skincare needs and enhancing their daily hygiene routines with high-quality, customized soap products.

CHAPTER SEVEN

MARKETING AND SELLING YOUR LIQUID SOAP

7.1. Branding Your Product

Branding your liquid soap product is essential for creating a distinct identity that resonates with your target audience. Effective branding not only differentiates your product from competitors but also builds trust, communicates quality, and encourages customer loyalty. Here's a comprehensive approach to branding your liquid soap product:

1. Define Your Brand Identity

- ✓ **Mission and Values**: Clarify your brand's purpose and core values. What values does your liquid soap promote, such as sustainability, natural ingredients, or community support?

- ✓ **Unique Selling Proposition (USP)**: Identify what sets your product apart from others in the market. Is it handmade, eco-friendly packaging, or specific skin benefits?

- ✓ **Target Audience**: Understand your ideal customers—seniors seeking gentle skincare, environmentally conscious consumers, or those interested in luxury pampering.

2. Develop a Brand Name and Logo

✓ **Name Selection**: Choose a memorable and relevant name for your liquid soap that reflects its benefits or target market. Ensure it's easy to pronounce and spell.

✓ **Logo Design**: Create a visually appealing logo that represents your brand's values and appeals to your target audience. Consider colors, fonts, and symbols that convey cleanliness, nature, or luxury.

3. Packaging Design

✓ **Packaging Material**: Select eco-friendly and functional packaging materials that align with your brand's sustainability goals.

✓ **Labeling**: Clearly communicate key information such as ingredients, benefits, and usage instructions. Use appealing visuals and fonts that match your brand aesthetic.

4. Brand Storytelling

- ✓ **Origin Story**: Share the inspiration behind your liquid soap product. Whether it's a family recipe, a commitment to natural ingredients, or a personal journey, storytelling creates emotional connections with consumers.

- ✓ **Customer Testimonials**: Highlight positive experiences and testimonials from satisfied customers to build credibility and trust.

5. Brand Voice and Messaging

- ✓ **Tone**: Determine the personality of your brand—friendly, authoritative, or nurturing—and maintain consistency in all communications.

- ✓ **Messaging**: Craft compelling messages that resonate with your target audience's needs and aspirations. Emphasize the benefits of using your liquid soap, such as gentle cleansing, moisturizing properties, or eco-consciousness.

6. Establish an Online Presence

- ✓ **Website**: Create a user-friendly website that showcases your liquid soap product, brand story, and purchasing options. Include an online store for seamless transactions.

✓ **Social Media**: Utilize platforms like Instagram, Facebook, or Pinterest to visually showcase your product, share skincare tips, and engage with your audience.

7. Marketing Strategies

✓ **Content Marketing**: Produce valuable content such as blog posts, tutorials, or skincare tips related to liquid soap use. Establish yourself as an expert in natural skincare or sustainable living.

✓ **Influencer Partnerships**: Collaborate with influencers or bloggers who align with your brand values to reach a wider audience.

✓ **Promotions and Discounts**: Offer introductory discounts, bundle deals, or seasonal promotions to attract new customers and encourage repeat purchases.

8. Customer Experience and Feedback

- ✓ **Customer Service**: Provide exceptional customer service, responding promptly to inquiries and resolving issues effectively.

- ✓ **Feedback Loop**: Encourage customer feedback through reviews, surveys, or social media interactions. Use insights to refine your product and marketing strategies.

9. Sustainability and Ethics

- ✓ **Environmental Responsibility**: Emphasize your commitment to sustainability through eco-friendly practices, packaging, and ingredient sourcing.

- ✓ **Ethical Practices**: Ensure transparency in your supply chain and manufacturing processes, promoting fair labor practices and cruelty-free testing.

10. Monitor and Adapt

- ✓ **Analytics**: Use analytics tools to track website traffic, sales trends, and customer demographics. Adjust your marketing strategies based on data insights to optimize performance.

✓ **Market Trends**: Stay informed about industry trends, consumer preferences, and competitor activities to stay relevant and competitive in the market.

Branding your liquid soap product involves crafting a compelling identity that resonates with your target audience, communicates value, and builds trust. By defining your brand identity, developing a memorable name and logo, creating appealing packaging, and engaging customers through storytelling and digital marketing, you can effectively differentiate your product in a competitive market. Implementing sustainable practices, prioritizing customer experience, and adapting to market feedback are key to establishing a successful brand presence and achieving long-term growth and profitability in selling your liquid soap.

7.2. Packaging and Labeling

Packaging and labeling play a crucial role in the presentation, protection, and promotion of your liquid soap product. Effective packaging not only attracts customers but also communicates essential information and ensures regulatory compliance. Here's a comprehensive approach to packaging and labeling your liquid soap:

1. Packaging Design

- ✓ **Functionality**: Choose packaging that is practical for storing and dispensing liquid soap, such as bottles with pump dispensers or squeeze bottles for easy use.

- ✓ **Material**: Opt for eco-friendly materials like recyclable plastic, glass, or biodegradable options to align with sustainable practices.

- ✓ **Aesthetic Appeal**: Design packaging that reflects your brand's identity and appeals to your target audience's preferences. Consider colors, shapes, and textures that convey cleanliness, luxury, or natural ingredients.

2. Labeling Requirements

- ✓ **Product Name**: Clearly display the name of your liquid soap product in a prominent font size that is easy to read.

✓ **Ingredients**: List all ingredients in descending order of predominance by weight. Include common names and indicate active ingredients.

✓ **Net Weight or Volume**: Specify the net weight (for solids) or net volume (for liquids) of the product in metric units (grams, milliliters, etc.).

✓ **Usage Instructions**: Provide clear directions for use, including how to dispense and apply the liquid soap.

✓ **Safety Information**: Include any necessary warnings or precautions, such as avoiding contact with eyes or keeping out of reach of children.

✓ **Manufacturer Information**: Display the name and address of the manufacturer, packer, or distributor. Include contact information for customer inquiries or feedback.

3. Designing Labels

✓ **Layout**: Organize label information in a clear and organized layout. Use bullet points or sections to distinguish different types of information (ingredients, usage, etc.).

✓ **Font and Colors**: Choose legible fonts and contrast colors for easy readability. Ensure text size is appropriate for the label size.

✓ **Brand Logo**: Incorporate your brand logo or symbol to reinforce brand recognition and identity.

✓ **Visual Elements**: Use graphics, icons, or imagery that complement your brand's theme or communicate product benefits (e.g., natural ingredients, moisturizing properties).

4. Regulatory Compliance

✓ **FDA Regulations**: Ensure compliance with FDA regulations for cosmetics, including ingredient labeling, claims substantiation, and safety testing requirements.

✓ **Allergen Information**: Clearly identify common allergens if present in the ingredients (e.g., nuts, soy, gluten).

✓ **Country-Specific Requirements**: Research and adhere to labeling requirements specific to your target market or country of distribution.

5. Sustainability Considerations

✓ **Environmentally Friendly**: Choose packaging materials that minimize environmental impact and promote recycling or composting.

✓ **Minimalist Design**: Opt for minimalist labeling to reduce material use and waste while maintaining essential information clarity.

6. Quality Assurance

✓ **Testing**: Conduct stability and compatibility testing to ensure packaging materials can safely contain and preserve liquid soap without leakage or contamination.

✓ **Feedback Mechanism**: Implement a system for gathering and addressing customer feedback regarding packaging functionality and design.

7. Brand Consistency

✓ **Consistent Branding**: Ensure packaging and labeling align with your overall brand identity, including tone, colors, and messaging.

✓ **Customer Engagement**: Use packaging as a tool for storytelling and engaging customers with your brand's mission, values, and product benefits.

8. Practical Tips

- ✓ **Prototyping**: Create prototypes of packaging and labels to visualize the final product and make adjustments as needed.

- ✓ **Batch Coding**: Include batch or lot numbers on labels for traceability and quality control purposes.

Packaging and labeling your liquid soap product involves thoughtful consideration of design, functionality, regulatory compliance, and brand representation. By creating attractive, informative, and environmentally responsible packaging, you can enhance product appeal, build customer trust, and effectively communicate the value of your liquid soap to your target audience. Through meticulous design, adherence to regulatory standards, and a commitment to sustainability, you can establish a strong brand presence and ensure a positive customer experience with your liquid soap product.

7.3. Setting Up an Online Store

Launching an online store requires careful planning and execution to create a seamless shopping experience for customers. From selecting an e-commerce platform to optimizing product listings, here's how to set up your online store for selling liquid soap:

1. Choose an E-commerce Platform

- ✓ **Platform Selection**: Evaluate e-commerce platforms such as Shopify, WooCommerce (WordPress), BigCommerce, or Etsy based on your budget, technical expertise, and customization needs.

- ✓ **Features**: Look for features like customizable templates, secure payment gateways, inventory management, and shipping options suitable for selling liquid soap products.

2. Create Your Store

- ✓ **Domain Name**: Register a domain name that reflects your brand and is easy for customers to remember.

- ✓ **Design**: Customize your store's theme or template to align with your brand identity. Use clean, intuitive navigation and a responsive design for mobile users.

✓ **Product Categories**: Organize liquid soap products into categories (e.g., moisturizing soaps, antibacterial soaps) to help customers find products quickly.

3. Product Listings

✓ **Product Descriptions**: Write compelling and informative descriptions for each liquid soap product. Highlight key features, ingredients, benefits, and usage instructions.

✓ **High-Quality Images**: Use high-resolution images that showcase the packaging, texture, and color of your liquid soap. Include multiple angles and close-ups for clarity.

✓ **Videos**: Consider creating product demonstration videos or tutorials to engage customers and demonstrate product usage.

4. Secure Payment Options

✓ **Payment Gateways**: Integrate secure payment gateways (e.g., PayPal, Stripe) to accept credit/debit cards, digital wallets, and other payment methods preferred by your target audience.

✓ **SSL Certificate**: Ensure your online store has an SSL certificate to encrypt customer data and provide a secure checkout experience.

5. Shipping and Fulfillment

✓ **Shipping Options**: Offer flexible shipping options (e.g., standard, expedited) with transparent pricing and delivery estimates.

✓ **Packaging**: Specify packaging requirements for shipping liquid soap products safely to prevent leaks or damage during transit.

6. Customer Experience

✓ **User Interface**: Optimize user experience (UX) with intuitive navigation, fast loading times, and a streamlined checkout process.

✓ **Customer Support**: Provide multiple channels for customer support, such as live chat, email, or a dedicated FAQ section to address common queries.

7. Marketing and Promotion

- ✓ **SEO Optimization**: Optimize product descriptions and store content for search engines to improve visibility and attract organic traffic.

- ✓ **Social Media Integration**: Integrate social media buttons and shareable product links to encourage customers to promote your products on social platforms.

- ✓ **Email Marketing**: Build an email list and send personalized campaigns with product updates, promotions, and customer testimonials to drive sales.

8. Legal and Compliance

- ✓ **Terms of Service**: Draft clear terms of service, including return policies, shipping terms, and disclaimers related to product use and liability.

- ✓ **Privacy Policy**: Create a privacy policy that complies with data protection regulations (e.g., GDPR, CCPA) and outlines how customer data is collected and used.

9. Analytics and Optimization

✓ **Analytics Tools**: Use e-commerce analytics tools (e.g., Google Analytics, platform-specific analytics) to track sales performance, customer behavior, and conversion rates.

✓ **Continuous Improvement**: Monitor metrics and customer feedback to identify areas for improvement in product offerings, marketing strategies, and user experience.

10. Launch and Promotion

✓ **Soft Launch**: Conduct a soft launch to test functionality, gather feedback, and make necessary adjustments before a full-scale launch.

✓ **Promotional Campaigns**: Plan promotional campaigns (e.g., launch discounts, limited-time offers) to generate initial buzz and attract early customers.

Setting up an online store for your liquid soap products involves strategic planning, attention to detail, and a focus on delivering a seamless shopping experience for customers. By choosing the right e-commerce platform, optimizing product listings, ensuring secure payments, and implementing effective marketing strategies, you can establish a strong online presence, attract customers, and drive sales. Continuously monitor performance metrics, gather customer feedback, and adapt your strategies to maximize growth and success in selling your liquid soap products online.

7.4. Marketing Strategies

Developing effective marketing strategies is crucial for promoting your liquid soap products, attracting customers, and increasing sales. Here's an extensive guide to help you implement successful marketing strategies:

Marketing strategies for your liquid soap products involve a mix of digital marketing, content creation, and customer engagement tactics to reach your target audience and drive conversions. Here's how to effectively market your liquid soap:

1. Identify Your Target Audience

- ✓ **Demographics**: Define the demographics of your ideal customers, such as age, gender, location, and income level.

✓ **Psychographics**: Understand their interests, values, lifestyles, and purchasing behaviors related to skincare and eco-friendly products.

2. Brand Positioning

✓ **Unique Selling Proposition (USP)**: Clearly communicate what sets your liquid soap apart from competitors. Highlight benefits such as natural ingredients, moisturizing properties, or sustainable packaging.

✓ **Brand Story**: Share the story behind your brand—whether it's a commitment to natural skincare, a family tradition, or a mission to reduce environmental impact.

3. Digital Marketing

✓ **Website Optimization**: Ensure your online store is user-friendly, mobile-responsive, and optimized for search engines (SEO) to attract organic traffic.

✓ **Content Marketing**: Create valuable content related to skincare tips, ingredient benefits, and soap-making tutorials to engage and educate your audience.

✓ **Email Campaigns**: Build an email list and send targeted campaigns with product updates, promotions, and customer testimonials to nurture leads and encourage repeat purchases.

4. Social Media Marketing

✓ **Platform Selection**: Choose social media platforms (e.g., Instagram, Facebook, Pinterest) based on where your target audience is most active.

✓ **Visual Content**: Use high-quality images, videos, and user-generated content to showcase your liquid soap products and demonstrate usage.

✓ **Influencer Partnerships**: Collaborate with influencers or micro-influencers who align with your brand values to reach their followers and build credibility.

5. Paid Advertising

✓ **PPC Ads**: Run pay-per-click (PPC) ads on search engines (Google Ads) and social media platforms to target specific keywords and demographics.

✓ **Social Media Ads**: Utilize targeted advertising options on platforms like Facebook Ads or Instagram Ads to reach a broader audience and drive traffic to your online store.

6. Promotions and Discounts

✓ **Launch Offers**: Offer introductory discounts or bundle deals for new customers to incentivize first-time purchases.

✓ **Seasonal Promotions**: Plan promotions around holidays, seasonal changes, or special events to capitalize on increased consumer spending.

7. Customer Engagement

✓ **Reviews and Testimonials**: Encourage satisfied customers to leave reviews and testimonials on your website and social media channels to build social proof.

✓ **Customer Loyalty Programs**: Implement loyalty programs or referral incentives to reward repeat customers and encourage word-of-mouth referrals.

8. Community Building

✓ **Online Forums and Groups**: Participate in relevant online forums, Facebook groups, or Reddit communities related to skincare or eco-friendly living to engage with potential customers.

✓ **Brand Partnerships**: Collaborate with complementary brands or local businesses for cross-promotions and co-branded campaigns to expand your reach.

9. Analytics and Optimization

✓ **Performance Tracking**: Use analytics tools to monitor the effectiveness of your marketing campaigns, track website traffic, and measure conversion rates.

✓ **A/B Testing**: Experiment with different ad creatives, messaging, and promotional offers to optimize campaign performance and maximize ROI.

10. Customer Feedback and Adaptation

- ✓ **Feedback Loop**: Gather and analyze customer feedback through surveys, reviews, and social media interactions to identify areas for improvement and adjust your marketing strategies accordingly.

- ✓ **Adaptation**: Stay agile and responsive to market trends, consumer preferences, and competitive landscape to maintain relevance and sustain growth.

Implementing effective marketing strategies for your liquid soap products involves understanding your target audience, establishing a strong brand presence, and leveraging digital channels to drive engagement and sales. By focusing on clear messaging, engaging content, strategic advertising, and customer-centric approaches, you can effectively promote your liquid soap products, build brand loyalty, and achieve long-term success in the competitive skincare market. Continuously monitor performance metrics, adapt your strategies based on insights, and prioritize customer satisfaction to foster sustainable growth and profitability for your liquid soap business.

7.4.1. Social Media Marketing

Social media marketing is a powerful tool for promoting your liquid soap products, engaging with your target audience, and driving sales. Here's an extensive guide on how to effectively leverage social media for marketing your liquid soap:

Social media platforms provide a dynamic environment to connect with potential customers, build brand awareness, and showcase the unique benefits of your liquid soap products. Here's how to create a successful social media marketing strategy:

1. Platform Selection

- ✓ **Identify Your Audience**: Choose social media platforms where your target audience is most active. Popular platforms for skincare products include Instagram, Facebook, Pinterest, and TikTok.

- ✓ **Platform Characteristics**: Understand each platform's strengths—visual content on Instagram, community engagement on Facebook, inspiration boards on Pinterest—to tailor your approach.

2. Profile Optimization

- ✓ **Profile Bio**: Write a compelling bio that highlights your brand's USP, key products, and a call-to-action (CTA) to visit your website or shop.

- ✓ **Profile Picture and Cover Photo**: Use high-quality images or your brand logo to create a professional and recognizable profile.

3. Content Strategy

- ✓ **Visual Content**: Share high-resolution images and videos that showcase your liquid soap products, ingredients, and packaging. Use lifestyle imagery to illustrate product benefits and usage scenarios.

- ✓ **Educational Content**: Create content that educates your audience about skincare benefits, ingredient transparency, and eco-friendly practices related to your liquid soap.

4. Engagement Tactics

- ✓ **Respond to Comments**: Engage with your audience by responding to comments, messages, and questions promptly. Encourage conversation and build relationships with potential customers.

✓ **User-Generated Content (UGC)**: Encourage customers to share their experiences with your liquid soap products through reviews, testimonials, and photos. Repost UGC to showcase social proof.

5. Influencer Partnerships

✓ **Identify Relevant Influencers**: Collaborate with influencers or micro-influencers in the skincare or eco-friendly niche who resonate with your brand values and target audience.

✓ **Partnership Campaigns**: Create sponsored content or influencer giveaways to reach a broader audience and build credibility through trusted recommendations.

6. Hashtag Strategy

✓ **Research Relevant Hashtags**: Use popular and niche hashtags related to skincare, natural ingredients, and liquid soap to increase visibility and attract targeted followers.

✓ **Create Branded Hashtags**: Develop unique hashtags specific to your brand or campaigns to encourage user engagement and track content related to your products.

7. Contests and Giveaways

- ✓ **Increase Engagement**: Host contests or giveaways that require participants to engage with your brand (e.g., liking, sharing, tagging friends) to expand reach and attract new followers.

- ✓ **Promote Product Trials**: Offer free samples or exclusive discounts to contest winners or participants, encouraging them to try and review your liquid soap products.

8. Paid Advertising

- ✓ **Targeted Ads**: Utilize paid advertising options on social media platforms (e.g., Facebook Ads, Instagram Ads) to target specific demographics, interests, and behaviors relevant to your target audience.

- ✓ **Retargeting Campaigns**: Implement retargeting ads to reach users who have previously visited your website or engaged with your social media content, encouraging them to complete a purchase.

9. Analytics and Optimization

✓ **Performance Tracking**: Use social media analytics tools to monitor key metrics such as engagement rate, reach, impressions, and conversions. Analyze data to optimize content strategy and ad campaigns.

✓ **Experimentation**: Test different content formats, posting schedules, and advertising strategies to identify what resonates best with your audience and drives the highest return on investment (ROI).

10. Community Building

✓ **Create Community Engagement**: Foster a sense of community by initiating discussions, sharing customer stories, and encouraging feedback and reviews.

✓ **Brand Advocacy**: Cultivate relationships with loyal customers who can become brand advocates, sharing their positive experiences and recommending your liquid soap products to their networks.

Social media marketing offers vast opportunities to promote your liquid soap products, engage with your audience, and build a loyal customer base. By leveraging platform-specific strategies, creating compelling content, engaging with influencers, and optimizing paid advertising, you can effectively increase brand visibility, drive traffic to your online store, and ultimately boost sales. Continuously monitor performance metrics, adapt your strategy based on insights, and prioritize authentic engagement to sustain long-term growth and success in marketing your liquid soap products through social media.

7.4.2. Craft Fairs and Local Markets

Craft fairs and local markets provide excellent opportunities to showcase and sell your liquid soap products directly to consumers, build brand awareness, and connect with your local community. Here's how to effectively leverage craft fairs and local markets as part of your marketing strategy:

Craft Fairs and Local Markets Marketing Strategy

Craft fairs and local markets offer a unique offline marketing channel where you can engage with potential customers face-to-face, receive immediate feedback, and build relationships. Here's how to make the most of these opportunities:

1. Research and Preparation

- ✓ **Event Selection**: Research local craft fairs, farmers' markets, and artisanal events in your area that attract your target audience—such as eco-conscious consumers or skincare enthusiasts.

- ✓ **Application Process**: Apply early and follow event guidelines for booth sizes, fees, and required permits or licenses.

2. Booth Setup

- ✓ **Eye-Catching Display**: Design an attractive booth display that showcases your liquid soap products effectively. Use branded signage, shelves, tablecloths, and lighting to create a visually appealing presentation.

✓ **Product Sampling**: Offer samples or testers of your liquid soap products to allow customers to experience the quality and fragrance firsthand.

3. Branding and Collateral

✓ **Branded Materials**: Create professional business cards, brochures, or flyers that highlight your brand story, product benefits, and contact information.

✓ **Signage**: Display clear signage with your brand name, logo, and product offerings to attract attendees from a distance.

4. Customer Engagement

✓ **Product Demonstrations**: Demonstrate how to use your liquid soap products and explain their benefits to potential customers.

✓ **Educational Content**: Share information about the ingredients, production process, and sustainability practices behind your liquid soap to educate and build trust with customers.

5. Promotions and Special Offers

✓ **Event Discounts**: Offer exclusive discounts or special promotions for attendees who make a purchase at the event.

✓ **Bundle Deals**: Create bundle deals or gift sets that encourage customers to purchase multiple products or try different variants of your liquid soap.

6. Collect Customer Feedback

✓ **Feedback Forms**: Provide feedback forms or surveys to gather insights about customer preferences, product satisfaction, and suggestions for improvement.

✓ **Email List**: Invite attendees to join your email list or follow your social media channels for future updates and promotions.

7. Networking and Collaboration

✓ **Connect with Other Vendors**: Network with fellow vendors and artisans at the event to explore collaboration opportunities, cross-promotions, or joint marketing efforts.

✓ **Local Partnerships**: Partner with local businesses or organizations to co-host events, sponsorships, or community initiatives that align with your brand values.

8. Follow-Up and Relationship Building

✓ **Customer Follow-Up**: Follow up with attendees after the event through personalized thank-you emails, special offers, or updates on new products.

✓ **Customer Loyalty**: Build relationships with repeat customers by offering loyalty rewards, referral incentives, or exclusive previews of upcoming products.

9. Brand Consistency

✓ **Consistent Messaging**: Maintain consistency in your brand messaging, storytelling, and visual identity across all marketing materials and interactions.

✓ **Customer Experience**: Prioritize excellent customer service and create memorable experiences that leave a positive impression on attendees.

10. Measure Success

✓ **Sales Tracking**: Keep track of sales metrics, such as total revenue, average transaction value, and popular products, to evaluate event success.

✓ **Feedback Analysis**: Review customer feedback and insights gathered during the event to identify areas for improvement and inform future marketing strategies.

Craft fairs and local markets offer valuable opportunities to promote your liquid soap products, engage with customers directly, and build brand awareness within your community. By preparing thoroughly, creating an inviting booth display, engaging with attendees through demonstrations and educational content, offering promotions, and following up with potential leads, you can maximize your presence at these events and drive sales. Incorporate these offline marketing strategies alongside your digital efforts to create a well-rounded marketing approach that strengthens your brand presence and supports long-term growth for your liquid soap business.

7.4.3. Collaborations and Partnerships

Collaborations and partnerships can significantly amplify your marketing efforts for liquid soap products by expanding your reach, enhancing credibility, and accessing new customer segments. Here's an extensive guide on how to leverage collaborations and partnerships effectively:

Collaborations and Partnerships for Marketing Your Liquid Soap Products

Collaborations and partnerships allow you to tap into complementary brands, influencers, and organizations to create mutually beneficial relationships that drive brand awareness, engagement, and sales. Here's how to strategize and execute successful collaborations:

1. Identify Strategic Partners

- ✓ **Complementary Brands**: Identify brands in related industries (e.g., skincare, eco-friendly products) whose values and target audience align with yours.

- ✓ **Influencers and Bloggers**: Collaborate with influencers or bloggers who have a strong following in the skincare, beauty, or sustainability niche.

- ✓ **Local Businesses**: Partner with local boutiques, spas, or wellness centers that share your target demographic and can promote your products to their customers.

2. Define Partnership Objectives

- ✓ **Marketing Goals**: Clarify your objectives, such as increasing brand visibility, reaching new markets, driving website traffic, or launching a new product line.

- ✓ **Mutual Benefits**: Outline what each partner will gain from the collaboration, whether it's exposure, content creation, cross-promotion, or access to new customers.

3. Collaboration Ideas

- ✓ **Co-Branded Products**: Create limited-edition or co-branded liquid soap products that combine your brand's expertise with the partner's unique offerings.

- ✓ **Content Collaboration**: Co-create blog posts, videos, or social media content that educates and entertains your shared audience about skincare tips, ingredient benefits, or sustainability practices.

- ✓ **Event Sponsorship**: Sponsor or co-host events, workshops, or webinars focused on skincare, wellness, or eco-conscious living, where you can showcase your liquid soap products.

4. Execution and Implementation

- ✓ **Agreements**: Draft a partnership agreement outlining responsibilities, timelines, promotional activities, and any financial arrangements.

- ✓ **Creative Assets**: Develop branded visuals, messaging, and promotional materials that maintain consistency across both brands and resonate with your target audience.

- ✓ **Launch Strategy**: Coordinate a joint marketing campaign to launch the collaboration, including social media teasers, email newsletters, and press releases to generate excitement.

5. Cross-Promotion and Outreach

- ✓ **Social Media Campaigns**: Share each other's content, tag partner brands in posts, and leverage influencers' reach to amplify your message and attract new followers.

- ✓ **Email Marketing**: Collaborate on email campaigns that introduce your products to each other's subscriber lists, offering exclusive discounts or incentives to drive conversions.

6. Measure and Evaluate

✓ **Performance Metrics**: Track key performance indicators (KPIs) such as engagement rates, website traffic, sales attributed to the collaboration, and social media follower growth.

✓ **Feedback**: Gather feedback from customers, influencers, and partners to assess the collaboration's impact, strengths, and areas for improvement.

7. Long-Term Relationship Building

✓ **Nurture Relationships**: Maintain open communication and foster a positive relationship with partners even after the collaboration ends.

✓ **Repeat Collaborations**: Explore opportunities for ongoing partnerships, seasonal promotions, or new product launches that continue to benefit both brands.

8. Legal Considerations

✓ **Contracts**: Ensure legal agreements cover intellectual property rights, confidentiality, liability, and termination clauses to protect both parties.

✓ **Compliance**: Adhere to advertising guidelines and regulatory requirements related to product claims, endorsements, and disclosures in collaborative campaigns.

9. Community Impact

✓ **Social Responsibility**: Align with partners on sustainable practices, ethical sourcing, and community initiatives that resonate with your shared values and appeal to conscious consumers.

10. Adaptation and Growth

✓ **Flexibility**: Stay adaptable to market trends, consumer preferences, and industry changes to seize new collaboration opportunities and maintain relevance.

Collaborations and partnerships are powerful strategies for marketing your liquid soap products, leveraging shared audiences, and amplifying brand visibility. By strategically identifying partners, setting clear objectives, executing creative campaigns, and measuring performance, you can create impactful collaborations that drive engagement, expand your customer base, and ultimately increase sales. Cultivate strong relationships with partners, prioritize mutual benefits, and continue to innovate to sustain long-term growth and success for your liquid soap business through strategic partnerships.

Conclusion

In conclusion, mastering the art of liquid soap making offers not only the satisfaction of creating unique, high-quality products but also the opportunity to delve into a craft that blends science with creativity. Throughout this book, we've explored the fundamental principles, detailed processes, and essential ingredients necessary to craft liquid soap that meets your standards of quality and sustainability.

From understanding the chemical reactions involved in saponification to mastering the techniques of formulation and customization, each step has been crafted to empower both beginners and seasoned soap makers alike. Safety precautions, equipment essentials, and troubleshooting tips have been highlighted to ensure a smooth and enjoyable soap-making journey.

HOMEMADE LIQUID SOAP MAKING

Beyond the technical aspects, we've delved into the artistic side of soap making—exploring the endless possibilities of fragrances, colors, and textures that allow you to personalize your creations. Whether you're crafting for personal use, gifting, or considering starting a business, the comprehensive knowledge shared here equips you with the confidence to experiment and innovate.

As you embark on your soap-making endeavors, remember that patience and practice are key. Embrace the process, learn from each batch, and celebrate your successes along the way. With dedication and creativity, you'll not only master the craft of liquid soap making but also discover a fulfilling and rewarding hobby or business venture that nourishes both body and soul.

May your soap-making adventures be filled with creativity, inspiration, and the joy of crafting something truly unique and beneficial. Here's to the artistry of liquid soap making and the endless possibilities it brings into your life.

THANKS FOR YOUR ATTENTION!!!

www.ingramcontent.com/pod-product-compliance
Lightning Source LLC
Chambersburg PA
CBHW051601250726
48653CB00004BA/1264